STRUCTURAL UNITS

OF

MEDICAL AND BIOLOGICAL TERMS

STRUCTURAL UNITS
OF
MEDICAL AND BIOLOGICAL TERMS

A Convenient Guide, in English, to The Roots,
Stems, Prefixes, Suffixes, and Other Combining
Forms Which Are The Building Blocks of Medical
and Related Scientific Words

By

J. E. SCHMIDT, M.D.

Medical Vocabulary Editor, MODERN MEDICINE

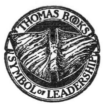

CHARLES C THOMAS • PUBLISHER

Springfield • Illinois • U.S.A.

Published and Distributed Throughout the World by
CHARLES C THOMAS • PUBLISHER
BANNERSTONE HOUSE
301-327 East Lawrence Avenue, Springfield, Illinois, U.S.A.
NATCHEZ PLANTATION HOUSE
735 North Atlantic Boulevard, Fort Lauderdale, Florida, U.S.A.

© 1969, by J. E. SCHMIDT
Library of Congress Catalog Card Number: 72-83838

With THOMAS BOOKS *careful attention is given to all details of
manufacturing and design. It is the Publisher's desire to present books
that are satisfactory as to their physical qualities and artistic possibilities
and appropriate for their particular use.* THOMAS BOOKS *will be true
to those laws of quality that assure a good name and good will.*

Printed in the United States of America
II-11

INTRODUCTION

The vocabulary of medicine is derived from numerous linguistic sources, such as Anglo-Saxon, French, Italian, Scandinavian, and Arabic, but the two chief sources, by far, are Greek and Latin.

From the Anglo-Saxon are derived mainly the vernacular anatomical terms, as *blood, finger, liver, mouth,* etc. From the French are derived such words as *bougie, chancre, tourniquet,* etc. A small group of words stem from Italian, *belladonna,* and *malaria,* for example. A few words, such as *scab* and *skin,* are from the Scandinavian, and there is a sprinkling of words from the German (*anlage, witzelsucht*), the Dutch (*sprue*), Chinese (*kaolin*), and Persian (*talc*).

As stated above, most of our vocabulary is derived from the Greek and Latin. And this is a happy philologic circumstance, primarily because the plastic roots of these languages are easily molded into useful combining forms. These classical languages provide convenient building blocks from which compound words of almost any length can be easily synthesized to meet the requirements of modern medical concepts. As a matter of fact, only a small portion of the total medical vocabulary consists of simple Greek and Latin words, as *meninx, pylorus, thorax* and *uterus.* The majority of the terms are compounds of two, three, or more combining forms, as *appendic-itis, chole-cyst-itis, thoraco-celo-schisis, hystero-vagino-entero-cele,* and *duodeno-chole-cyst-os-tomy.*

There are several kinds of combining forms or structural units. The more primitive or undifferentiated units are known as *stems* or *roots,* as *morph-* in *morph-o-logy.* (For our purpose, stems and roots may be regarded as having the same value.) A stem or root carries a specific idea, as *form* in the case of *morph-;* but bare roots or stems, like loose bricks, are seldom functional. To make them functional, they must be provided with one or more appendages which serve as links for the union with other combining forms.

A stem or root with its appendages may be regarded as a *differentiated combining form,* which, anatomically, may be compared to a nerve cell with its axon and dendrite. Thus, *morph-* in its differentiated and usable form appears as *morpho-.* The

v

appendage *o*, which converts *morph-* into *morpho-*, may be envisioned as a linguistic or verbal cement, a kind of mortar which joins the building blocks into a compact word.

Certain combining forms occur habitually at the beginning of words, i.e., they precede the concept-carrying stems or roots. Such forms are known as *prefixes*. Thus, *sub-* in *sub-normal* is a prefix. A prefix may consist of only one letter or one syllable, as the *a* in *a-mnesia, a-menorrhea,* or the *sub-* in *sub-scapular*. It may consist of more than one syllable, as *hy-po-* in *hypo-tension,* or of a modified word, as in *utero-sacral*.

Combining forms occurring at the end of a word are known as *suffixes*. Suffixes are composed of one or more letters or syllables and generally carry no specific meanings; however, they bear abstract qualities. Thus, the suffix *-ia* is used to form *names of diseases, biological classes,* etc., as in *pneumon-ia, hemophil-ia,* and *Mammal-ia*. Some suffixes form nouns denoting *character, condition,* etc., as *-icity* in *eccentr-icity, pathogen-icity,* etc.

A number of suffixes form nouns designating an *act, process* or *state,* as *-ion* in *incis-ion, lacerat-ion,* etc. A few suffixes denote *a person engaged in a given occupation,* as *-ist* in *gynecolog-ist, chem-ist*. Other suffixes carry the concept of *pertaining to, or of the nature of,* etc., as *-ive* in *suppurat-ive, ulcerat-ive, refract-ive,* etc.

The vast majority of the medical combining forms are composed of stems and roots, and more importantly, of their modified or differentiated forms, which carry specific meanings, as *patho-* (in *pathology*), *hyster-* (*hysterectomy*), *hemato-* (*hematopoiesis*), etc.

This *Dictionary of Structural Units* deals with all types of medical combining forms, but it is concerned mainly with the "bread and butter" units which carry specific meanings and contribute to the formation of all current and useful medical terms. The book gives the reader not only the stems and roots, which in their unmodified forms can be useful only to the expert, but also the differentiated and functional forms, complete with the necessary appendages or links. These completely organized forms illustrate clearly the minute anatomy of words and can easily be brought together, like so many boxcars, to form meaningful and complex medical terms.

Moreover, the combining forms or structural units in this book are arranged alphabetically on the basis of their meanings in English. This plan enables the reader to find the needed combining forms quite easily by looking under the concepts which they convey. Thus, if the reader wishes to compound a word meaning inflammation of the appendix, (assuming that such a word did not exist) he would look under *appendix* and there find the combining form *appendic-*; he would then look under *inflammation* and find the unit *-itis*. By combining the two structural units at their linkage points, the reader would form the word *appendicitis.*

Each entry in the book is treated exhaustively in accordance with a formula which divides the entry into three major parts. The first part lists one or more words expressing the meaning, in English, of the combining forms treated in the entry. This is the part the reader looks for first. Thus, the combining forms *cardi-* and *cardio-* will, quite logically, be found under *heart.* Since many combining forms are used in more than one sense, the initial clue (in this case *heart*) is often followed by words expressing related ideas (in the present example *cardiac sphincter of the stomach*).

The second part of the entry indicates the language from which the combining forms are derived and gives the complete classical word (in this example *kardia*) from which they are enucleated. Following this, the entry presents the actual and functional combining forms (in this case *cardi-* and *cardio-*).

The third part of the entry illustrates, by means of numerous examples, the manner in which the combining forms are linked or joined to produce compound words. In these copious examples, the structural unit under discussion is separated by a hyphen from the rest of the compound word to further elucidate the architecture of the medical vocabulary. Each example is also followed by a definition of the complete word, which perfects the understanding of the semantic contribution of the particular combining form.

To summarize, the purpose of this dictionary is to provide the reader with an easily understandable dissection of the medical vocabulary, to offer thousands of ready-to-use medical combining forms, and to illustrate by means of copious examples the semantic values of the various structural elements and the manner in which they are joined to form compound words.

Because the material is arranged alphabetically on the basis of the meanings or medical concepts, the user of the book can readily find the required combining forms for the synthesis of such new words as he may need. This reference book will, therefore, be especially valuable to medical researchers and medical authors who often need new terms with which to describe medical discoveries, new methods and ideas, and a variety of previously unrecorded medical phenomena.

STRUCTURAL UNITS

OF

MEDICAL AND BIOLOGICAL TERMS

A

abdomen (belly).

> (L. *abdomen,* belly; genit. *abdominis*) abdomin-; abdomino-.
> *Ex*: abdomin-al (pertaining to the abdomen); abdomin-algia (pain in the abdomen); abdomino-scopy (examination of the abdomen, especially by endoscopy); abdomino-thoracic (pertaining to the abdomen and the thorax).

abdomen (belly).

> (Gr. *koilia,* belly) celi-; celio-.
> *Ex*: celi-ac (pertaining to the abdomen); celi-algia (pain in the abdomen); celio-centesis (puncture of the abdominal wall); celio-scope (instrument to examine interior of abdomen).

abdomen (belly; anterior aspect).

> (L. *venter,* belly) ventr-; ventri-; ventro-.
> *Ex*: ventr-ad (toward the ventral side or aspect); ventri-cornu (the anterior cornu of the spinal cord); ventro-fixation (the fixation of the uterus to the anterior abdominal wall).

abdominal wall. See under *flank.*

abnormal. See under *beside.*

abnormal condition. See under *process.*

above (higher; over; excessive).

> (L. *super,* above) super-.
> *Ex*: super-alimentation (excessive feeding); super-natant (situated above the surface of a fluid); super-numerary (excessive in number); super-sonic (having a speed above that of sound).

above (over; higher).

> (L. *supra,* above) supra-.
> *Ex*: supra-clavicular (above the clavicle); supra-condylar (above a condyle); supra-mastoid (above the mastoid process); supra-pubic (above the pubic arch); supra-renal (above the kidney). See also *excessive.*

absence of. See under *without.*

accept. See under *receive.*

accessory to. See under *beside.*

ache. See under *pain.*

acid (sour).

> (Gr. *oxys,* acid) oxy-.
> *Ex*: oxy-rygmia (the eructation of acid or sour material); oxy-pathy (poisoning by an acid).

1

acid (sour).

    (L. *acidus,* sour) -acid-; acidi-; acido-.

    Ex: hyper-acid-ity (excessive acidity); hypo-acidity; acidi-fier (a substance which imparts or increases acidity); acidi-meter (a device to measure the amount of acid present); acido-philic (readily stained by acid dyes); acido-resistant (resisting decolorization by acids).

acid (vinegar).

    (L. *acetum,* vinegar) acet-; aceto-.

    Ex: acet-ic (pertaining to vinegar); acet-aldehyde (an aldehyde of vinegar or acetic acid); acet-anilid (a compound of aniline and acetic acid); Aceto-bacter (a genus of microorganisms capable of producing vinegar).

across (on other side; through; beyond).

    (L. *trans,* across) trans-.

    Ex: trans-aortic (through the aorta); trans-iliac (across the ilia); trans-pleural (performed through the pleura); trans-uranium (beyond uranium).

acute.   See under *sharp.*

adhesion. See under *immobility.*

adjacent. See under *beside.*

affinity. See under *loving.*

after (following; behind; later).

    (L. *post,* after) post-.

    Ex: post-adolescent (occurring after adolescence); post-nasal (behind or in the back of the nose); post-partum (after childbirth); post-traumatic (occurring after an injury).

after (post; next).

    (Gr. *meta,* after) met-; meta-.

    Ex: meta-chronous (occurring after or at a later time); meta-pyretic (occurring after a fever); meta-tarsus (the part of the foot next to the tarsus).

again (repetition; backward)

    (Gr. *palin,* again) pali-; palin-.

    Ex: pali-kinesia (abnormal repetition of a movement); pali-lalia (abnormal repetition of a word or words); palin-genesis (the appearance of an old characteristic in a new generation).

again. See under *back.*

against (opposed; contrary; opposite).

(L. *contra,* against) contra-.
Ex: contra-ceptive (opposed to conception); contra-fissure (fracture in a place opposite the site of the blow); contra-lateral (pertaining to the opposite side).

against (opposite; reverse; opposed to; instead).

(Gr. *anti,* against) ant-; anti-.
Ex: ant-agonist (a muscle acting in opposition); ant-acid; anti-biotic; anti-coagulant (a substance which opposes coagulation); anti-histamine; anti-toxin (a substance which opposes or neutralizes a toxin).

aged. See under *old age.*

air (gas).

(Gr. *physa,* bellows; *physaein,* to blow) -phys-; physo-.
Ex: physo-cele (a sac or space filled with gas); physo-metra (presence of air in the uterus); em-phys-ema; physo-salpinx (presence of air or gas in a uterine tube).

air (gas; atmosphere).

(Gr. *aer,* air; genit. *aeros*) -aer-; aeri-; -aero-.
Ex: aer-emia (the presence of air in the blood); an-aero-be (a microorganism which lives in the absence or air or oxygen); aer-ated (charged with or exposed to air); aeri-ferous (bearing or conveying air); aero-biology (the science dealing with the distribution of organisms by air); aero-genesis (production or air or gas).

air (gas; respiration).

(Gr. *pneuma,* air) pneum-; pneuma-; pneumato-; pneumo-.
Ex: pneum-arthrosis (the presence of air or any gas in a joint cavity); pneuma-type (the moisture deposit on a glass surface from the exhaled air); pneumato-cele (a sac or swelling containing gas); pneumo-derma (the presence of gas in the subcutaneous tissue). See also *lung.*

alike. See under *equal.*

alive (living).

(L. *vivus*, alive) vivi-; vivo-.

Ex: vivi-dialysis (dialysis through a living membrane); vivi-parous (giving birth to living young); vivi-section; vivo-sphere (the region composed of the upper surface of the earth and the lower portion of the atmosphere where life exists).

all (every; universal).

(Gr. *pan*, all; genit. *pantos*) pan-; pant-; panto-.

Ex: pan-angiitis (inflammation of all the coats of a blood vessel); pan-carditis (inflammation of all three layers of the heart wall); pant-algia (pain in all parts of the body); panto-scopic (pertaining to both near and far vision).

all (everywhere; unrestricted; universal).

(L. *omnis*, all) omni-.

Ex: omni-vorous (eating all kinds of food); omni-cellular (pertaining to all types of cell); omni-chromopsia (the ability to perceive all colors).

almost. See under *under.*

aloft. See under *high.*

alone. See under *one.*

altered. See under *changed.*

alveolar process. See under *alveolus.*

alveolus (socket; small cavity).

(L. *alveolus*, small hollow) alveol-; alveolo-.

Ex: alveol-itis (inflammation of an alveolus); alveolo-dental (pertaining to an alveolus and a tooth); alveolo-plasty (plastic surgery on an alveolus or alveolar process).

among. See under *between.*

angle.

(Gr. *gonia*, angle) goni-; gonio-.

Ex: gonio-craniometry (the measurement of the anatomical angles of the cranium); gonio-meter (an instrument used in measuring angles); gonio-scopy (examination of the angle of the eye).

animal (beast).

(Gr. *zoon*, animal) zo-; zoo-.

Ex: zo-anthropy (belief by patient that he is an animal); zoodermic (pertaining to the skin of an animal); zoo-logy; zoo-philism (love for animals); zoo-toxin (a toxin produced by an animal).

anion. See under *ion.*

ankle bone. See under *talus.*

ankylosis. See under *immobility.*

another. See under *other.*

anterior. See under *before* and *front.*

anterior aspect. See under *abdomen.*

antrum (sinus; cavity).

(Gr. *antron,* a cave; L. *antrum*) -antr-; antro-.

Ex: antr-odynia (pain in an antrum); antro-stomy (formation of an opening in an antrum); antro-scopy (inspection of an antrum).

anvil-shaped. See under *incus.*

apparent. See under *visible.*

appearance. See under *face.*

appetite (desire; striving).

(Gr. *orexis,* appetite) orex-; -orex; orexi-.

Ex: an-orex-ia (lack of appetite for food); orexi-fugic (diminishing the appetite); orexi-genic (stimulating the appetite).

appreciation. See under *knowledge.*

area. See under *place.*

arm (upper extremity).

(Gr. *brachion,* arm) brachi-; brachio-.

Ex: brachi-algia (pain in an arm); brachio-cephalic (pertaining to the arm and head); brachio-tomy (obstetrical removal of an arm).

armpit (axilla).

(Gr. *maschale,* armpit) maschal-; maschalo-.

Ex: maschal-adenitis (inflammation of the axillary lymph nodes); maschal-oncus (a tumor or mass in the axilla); maschalo-lagnia (sexual craving for the female axilla).

armpit. See also under *axilla.*

aroma. See under *odor.*

around (surrounding).

(L. *circum,* around) circum-.

Ex: circum-anal (surrounding the anus); circum-corneal
(surrounding the cornea); circum-ference (outer margin of
a round object).

around (surrounding; encircling).

(Gr. *peri,* around) peri-.

Ex: peri-adenitis (inflammation of the tissue surrounding a
gland); peri-appendicular (surrounding the appendix); peri-
articular (around a joint); peri-osteum (layer of tissue surrounding a bone).

arrangement (orientation; order).

(Gr. *taxis,* arrangement) taxo-; -taxis.

Ex: taxo-nomy (the arrangement or classification of organisms); photo-taxis (orientation of an organism in response to
light); chemo-taxis (orientation in response to a chemical stimulus).

arrest.   See under *standing.*

artery.

(L. *arteria,* artery, windpipe) arter-; arteri-; arterio-.

Ex: arter-itis (inflammation of an artery); arteri-al (pertaining
to an artery); arteri-ectasis (abnormal dilatation of an artery);
arteri-ectomy (excision of a portion of an artery); arterio-plasty
(a plastic operation on an artery); arterio-spasm (a spasm
of an artery).

articulation (joint).

(L. *articulatio,* articulation) -articul-.

Ex: articul-ar (pertaining to an articulation); sub-articular (below an articulation); articul-ator (a joint-like device).

artificial structure.   See under *prosthesis.*

aspect.   See under *face.*

atmosphere.   See under *air.*

atrium (auricle).

(Gr. *atrion,* hall, chamber; L. *atrium*) atri-; atrio-.

Ex: atri-al (pertaining to an atrium); atrio-megaly (enlargement of an atrium); atrio-ventrivular (pertaining to an atrium
and a ventricle).

attachment. See under *fixation.*
auditory tube. See under *tube.*
auricle. See under *ear.*
aversion. See under *fear* and *hate.*
away from. See under *from* and *out.*
axilla (armpit).
> (L. *axilla,* armpit) -axill-; -axillary; axillo-.
> *Ex*: axill-ary (pertaining to or involving the armpit); intra-axillary (situated in the armpit); axillo-thoracic (pertaining to the armpit and the chest wall).

axis (axle).
> (L. *axis;* Gr. *axon*) ax-; axi-; axio-.
> *Ex*: axi-fugal (moving away from an axis); oxi-petal (moving toward an axis); axio-buccal (pertaining to the axial and buccal walls of a tooth cavity).

B

bacillus (rod).
> (L. *bacillus,* small rod or stick) bacill-; bacilli-; bacillo-.
> *Ex*: bacill-ary (pertaining to bacilli); bacillemia; bacilli-cide (agent destructive to bacilli); bacillo-phobia.

back (backwards; again).
> (L.) re-.
> *Ex*: re-tract (to draw back); re-cidivism (a turning back to crime); re-generate (to generate again); re-pellent (an agent that drives back).

back (posterior; dorsum).
> (L. *dorsum,* back) dors-; dorsi-; dorso-.
> *Ex*: dors-ad (toward the back); dorsi-flexion (backward flexion, as of the foot); dorso-lateral (pertaining to the back and the side). See also *backward.*

back of body (back part).
> (Gr. *noton,* back) not-; noti-; noto-.
> *Ex*: not-odynia (pain in the back); noti-form (shaped like the back); campto-not-ia (condition of having a bent back); noto-chord.

back part. See under *back of body*.

backward (back; behind).

  (L. *retro,* backward) retro-.

  Ex: retro-auricular (behind an auricle); retro-cession (a displacement backward); retro-clavicular (behind the clavicle).

backward (behind; in the back; back).

  (Gr. *opisthen,* at the back) opisth-; opistho-.

  Ex: opisth-enar (the back of the hand); opistho-comial (wearing the hair long in the back); opisth-otic (behind the ear); opistho-gnathic (having a receding jaw); opistho-tonos (a form of tetanic spasm); opistho-poreia (a disorder manifested by walking backward).

bacterium (rod, staff).

  (Gr. *bakterion,* small rod) bacter-; bacteri-; bacterio-.

  Ex: bacter-emia (presence of bacteria in the blood); bactericidal (destructive to bacteria); bacterio-logy.

bad (ill; mean; deformed).

  (Gr. *kakos,* bad) cac-; caco-.

  Ex: cac-hexia (bad health and malnutrition); cac-odontia (bad teeth); caco-geusia (bad taste); cac-osmia (bad odor). See also *improper.*

bad odor. See under *stench*.

ball (sphere; globe; drop).

  (L. *globus,* ball; *globulus,* small ball) glob-; globul-; globuli-; globulo-.

  Ex: glob-ose (spherical); globuli-cidal (destructive to red blood corpuscles); globul-in; globulin-emia (presence of globulin in the blood); globulo-lytic (destructive to red blood cells).

band. See under *ligament*.

bare. See under *nude*.

base (bottom).

  (L. *fundus,* bottom) fund-; fundi-; fundo-; fundu-.

  Ex: fund-ectomy (excision of the base of an organ); fundo-plication (plication of the fundus of the stomach around esophagus); anti-fundic (opposite the fundus); fundu-scope (instrument for examining the fundus of the eye).

beak (beak-like structure).

(L. *rostrum,* beak) rostr-; rostri-.

Ex: rostr-ate (provided with a rostrum); rostri-form (shaped like a beak); rostr-al (pertaining to a rostrum or beak); rostr-ad (toward a rostrum).

beam. See under *ray.*

bear child (bring forth; give birth).

(L. *parere,* bring forth) -par-; -para.

Ex: par-ity (status of a woman with regard to her having borne children); par-ous (designating a woman who has borne one or more children); nulli-para (a woman who has never borne a child); multi-para (a woman who has borne two or more children in two or more pregnancies).

bearing (bearer; motion; direction).

(Gr. *pherein,* to bear) -phor-; -phora; -phore; -phoresis; -phoria; phoro-; -phorous; -phorus.

Ex: eu-phor-ous (marked by euphoria); Plasmodio-phora (a genus of parasitic organisms); gono-phore (a structure which carries reproductive cells, as a uterine tube); cata-phoresis (introduction of a medicinal substance into a tissue by the use of an electric field); eso-phoria (a turning of the eye inward, toward the nose); phoro-meter (an instrument to measure phorias); phos-phorous (having phosphorescence); phos-phorus (a substance marked by phosphorescence).

beast. See under *animal.*

bed (bedside; horizontal posture; lying).

(Gr. *kline,* bed) clin-; clinic-; clino-.

Ex: clin-ician (expert in clinical or bedside medicine); clinic (bedside instruction); clino-mania (abnormal desire to lie in bed); clino-therapy (treatment by rest in bed).

bee. See under *honey.*

before (in front of; occurring before).

(Gr. *pro,* before) pro-.

Ex: pro-cephalic (pertaining to the front part of the head; in front of the head); pro-chondral (preceding the formation of cartilage); pro-nucleus (the structure from which a nucleus is formed).

before (prior; earlier; anterior; in front).

(L. *prae,* before) pre-.

Ex: pre-cordial (pertaining to the region in front of the heart); pre-medical (prior to the regular medical courses); pre-patent (before becoming evident); pre-vertebral (in front of a vertebra).

before (prior; in front; forward).

(L. *ante,* before) ante-.

Ex: ante-cubital (in front of the elbow); ante-febrile (before the onset of fever); ante-partum (before labor); ante-natal (before birth); ante-location (a forward displacement).

beget. See under *produce.*

beginning. See under *primitive.*

behind. See under *after, backward,* and *posterior.*

being. See under *existence.*

belly. See under *abdomen.*

below. (beneath; underneath).

(L. *infra,* beneath) infra-.

Ex: infra-glenoid (below the glenoid cavity); infra-patellar (below the patella); infra-red (below the red end of the spectrum).

below. See under *beneath* and *under.*

bend (curve; flex).

(L. *flectere,* to bend; *flexus,* bent) -flect-; -flex-.

Ex: genu-flect (bend the knee); retro-flex-ion (a bending backward of an organ, as the uterus).

beneath (less than normal; under; below).

(Gr. *hypo,* under) hypo-.

Ex: hypo-acidity (presence of less than the normal amount of acid); hypo-dermic (applied or injected beneath the skin); hypo-mastia (a less than normal development of the breasts); hypo-tension (blood pressure which is below normal).

beneath. See under *below* and *under.*

bent (crooked; curved; looped).

(Gr. *ankylos,* crooked) ankylo-; ankyl-.

Ex: ankyl-osis (immobility and crookedness of a joint); ankylo-glossia (the condition of tongue-tie).

beside (adjacent; beyond; accessory to; against; apart from; abnormal; resembling).

(Gr. *para,* beside) par-; para-.

Ex: para-appendicitis (inflammation of the tissues adjacent to the appendix); para-blepsia (abnormal vision); para-chromatism (abnormal perception of colors); para-cyesis (a pregnancy outside of or beyond the uterus); para-hemophilia (a condition resembling hemophilia); para-medical (accessory to medicine); para-thyroid (situated beside or adjacent to the thyroid gland); par-onychia (inflammation of the tissue adjacent to the nail).

beside. See under *near.*

between (among; mutual; mutually).

(L. *inter,* between) inter-.

Ex: inter-articular (between the articular surfaces of bones); inter-clavicular (between the clavicles); inter-gluteal (between the gluteal muscles).

beyond (excessive).

(L. *ultra,* beyond) ultra-.

Ex: ultra-microscopic (beyond the vision through an ordinary microscope); ultra-sonic (beyond the range of perception by the human ear); ultra-violet (beyond the violet end of the spectrum).

beyond. See under *across, beside,* and *outside of.*

big. See under *large.*

bile (biliary).

(Gr. *chole,* bile) chol-; chole-; cholo-.

Ex: chol-agogue (agent which stimulates flow of bile); cholecyst (gallbladder); chole-poiesis (formation of bile); cholochrome (biliary pigment).

bile (gall).

(L. *bilis,* bile) bili-.

Ex: bili-ary (pertaining to bile); bili-rubin (a reddish bile pigment); bili-verdin (a green bile pigment).

bile duct.

(Gr. *chole,* bile; *angeion,* vessel) cholang-; cholangi-; cholangio-.

Ex: cholangi-ectasis (dilatation of a bile duct); cholangio-enterostomy (anastomosis of a bile duct with the intestine); cholangi-oma (tumor of a bile duct); cholang-itis (inflammation of a bile duct).

bile duct, common.

(Gr. *choledochos,* containing bile) choledoch-; choledocho-.

Ex: choledoch-ectomy (excision of the common bile duct); choledoch-itis (inflammation of the common bile duct); choledocho-stomy (formation of an opening in the common bile duct).

biliary calculus. See under *gallstone.*

billion. See under *gigantic.*

bird (birds).

(Gr. *ornis,* bird; genit. *ornithos*) ornith-; ornitho-.

Ex: ornith-osis (a disease of birds); ornitho-logy (the study of birds); ornitho-myzous (parasitic on birds); ornitho-phobia (fear of birds).

birth (nativity; descent).

(L. *nasci,* to be born; pp. *natus*) nat-; nati-; -natia.

Ex: nat-al (pertaining to birth); pre-nat-al (before birth); nati-mortality; pro-natia (premature birth).

bitter.

(Gr. *pikros,* bitter) picr-; picro-.

Ex: picr-ageusia (inability to preceive a bitter taste); picro-geusia (an abnormal sensation of a bitter taste); picro-carmine (a stain containing picric acid).

black (melanin).

(Gr. *melas,* black) melas-; melani-; melano-.

Ex: melan-emia (presence of black pigment in the blood); melani-ferous (containing or bearing melanin); melano-phore (a cell containing melanin).

bladder.

(L. *vesica,* bladder) -vesic-; vesico-.

Ex: vesic-al (pertaining to the bladder); retro-vesic-al (behind the bladder); vesico-abdominal (pertaining to the bladder and the abdomen); vesico-tomy (incision into the bladder).

bladder (cyst; sac; bag; pouch).

(Gr. *kystis,* sac) cyst-; cysti-; cystido-; cysto-.

Ex: cyst-atrophia (atrophy of the bladder); cyst-ectomy (excision of a cyst; excision of the bladder); cystido-trachelotomy (incision of the neck of the bladder); cyst-itis; cysto-gram (an x-ray picture of the bladder); cysto-lith (a calculus of the bladder).

blister (vesicle; pustule).

(Gr. *phlyktaina,* a blister) phlycten-; phlycteno-.

Ex: phlycten-ar (pertaining to phlyctenae); phlycten-oid (resembling phlyctenae); phlycten-osis (a condition marked by the presence of phlyctenae); phlycten-ule (a small phlyctena); phlycteno-therapy.

blister. See under *vesicle.*

blood.

(Gr. *haima,* blood; genit. *haimatos*) hem-; hema-; hemat-; hemato-; hemo-; -emia.

Ex: hem-angioma (a tumor composed of young blood vessels); hem-angiectasis (abnormal dilatation of blood vessels); hem-agglutinin (an antibody which causes agglutination of red blood cells); hema-cytometer (an instrument used in counting blood cells); hemat-emesis (the vomiting of matter containing blood); hemat-uria (the discharge of urine containing blood); hemato-poiesis (the formation of blood cells); hemo-globin; hemo-lysin (a substance which disintegrates red blood cells and liberates the hemoglobin). an-emia; septic-emia (presence of pathogenic microorganisms in the blood).

blood.

(L. *sanguis,* blood; genit. *sanguinis*) sangui-; sanguin-; sanguino-.

Ex: sangui-colous (living in the blood); sangui-ferous (conveying blood); sanguin-eous (pertaining to blood); sanguino-poietic (producing blood).

blood platelet. See under *platelet.*

blood serum. See under *serum.*

blood vessel. See under *vessel.*

blow. See under *paralysis.*

blue (cyanic acid).

(Gr. *kyanos,* blue) cyan-; cyani-; cyano-.

Ex: cyan-ate (a salt of cyanic acid); cyano-phil (staining readily with blue dyes); cyan-opsin (a visual bluish pigment).

body (body build).

(Gr. *soma,* body; genit. *somatos*) som-; somat-; somatico-; somato-.

Ex: som-asthenia (weakness of the body); somat-esthesia (the feeling of having a body); somatico-visceral (pertaining to the body and the viscera); somato-pleure (the body wall of the embryo).

bone (bone tissue; os).

(L. *os,* bone; genit. *ossis*) oss-; -ossi-; osseo-.

Ex: osseo-cartilaginous (composed of both bone and cartilage); osseo-sonometry (the scientific measurement of the degree of conduction of sound through bone); ossi-fication (the formation of bone, as from cartilage).

bone (bone tissue; osteon).

(Gr. *osteon,* a bone) ost-; oste-; osteo-.

Ex: oste-algia (pain in a bone); ost-ectomy (excision of a bone or a part thereof); oste-itis (inflammation of a bone); osteo-arthritis; osteo-chondroma (a tumor of bone and cartilage); ex-ost-osis (an outgrowth from the surface of a bone); en-ost-osis (an outgrowth from the internal surface of a bone).

bone of finger or toe. See under *phalanx.*

bone, small. See under *ossicle.*

both (both sides; double).

(Gr. *amphi,* on both sides) amphi-; ampho-.

Ex: amphi-bious (living both on land and in water); amphi-bolic (pertaining to both catabolism and anabolism); amphi-celous (having a concave surface on both sides); ampho-philic (taking the stain of both acid and basic dyes).

bottom. See under *base.*

brain (encephalon).

(Gr. *enkephalos,* brain) encephal-; encephali-; encephalo-.

Ex: encephal-algia (pain in the head or brain); encephalitis; encephalo-pathy (disease of the brain).

branch (ramus).

(L. *ramus,* branch) rami-; ram-.

Ex: rami-fication (a branching out); rami-section (the cutting of a branch or branches); ram-itis (inflammation of a root); ram-ose (having several branches).

branch of medicine. See under *science of.*

break (breakdown; fracture).

(Gr. *klasis,* break) -clas-; -clasis.

Ex: histo-clas-tic (breaking down tissues); odonto-clasis (fracture of a tooth); osteoclasis; dia-clasis (surgical fracture of a bone).

break (fracture).

(L. *frangere,* break; *fractus,* broken) fract-; fracto-; fractur-.

Ex: fract-ion (part broken off); fracto-cumulus (mass of ragged clouds torn from a cumulus); dif-fract-ion (the breaking up of a ray of light into its constituent parts); fractur-ography (the taking of x-ray pictures of a fractured bone).

break (rupture; bursting).

(Gr. *rhexis,* a bursting) -rrhexis.

Ex: onycho-rrhexis (a breaking of a nail); arterio-rrhexis (a rupture of an artery); tricho-rrhexis (brittleness of the hair).

breast (mammary gland).

(L. *mamma,* breast) mamm-; mamma-; mammi-; mammo-.

Ex: mamm-ectomy (surgical removal of a breast); mamma-plasty (a plastic operation on a breast); mamm-form (shaped like a breast); mammo-tropic (stimulating the breast).

breast (mammary gland).

(Gr. *mastos,* breast) mast-; masto-.

Ex: mast-algia (pain in the breast); mast-ectomy (surgical removal of a breast); mast-itis (inflammation of the breast); masto-pathy (any disease of the breast); masto-plasty (a plastic operation on a breast).

breast

(Gr. *mazos,* breast) -maz-; mazo-.

Ex: maz-odynia (pain in a breast); mazo-pexy (the fixation of a pendulous breast); mazo-plasia (a degenerative hyperplasia of the breast).

breastbone. See under *sternum.*

breathe (breath).

(L. *halare,* to breathe) -hal-; halit-.

Ex: ex-hal-ation (a breathing out); halit-us (expelled breath); halit-osis (unpleasant breath).

breathe (breathing; respiration).

(Gr. *pnein,* to breathe) -pnea; pneo-.

Ex: dys-pnea (difficult breathing); a-pnea (suspension of breathing); tachy-pnea (rapid breathing); pneo-meter (an instrument used to measure the air exchange in respiration).

breathing (breathe).

(L. *spirare,* to breathe) -spir-; -spirat-; -pir-; spiro-.

Ex: in-spir-ation (a breathing in); ex-pir-ation; re-spirat-or (an apparatus used to administer artificial respiration); spiro-meter (an apparatus used to measure the air inhaled and exhaled).

breathing. See under *respiration.*

bring forth. See under *bear child.*

brittle. See under *fragile.*

broad. See under *wide.*

bronchiole (bronchioles).

(L. *bronchiolus,* fine air passage) bronchiol-.

Ex: bronchiol-ectasis (dilatation of bronchioles); bronchiol-itis (inflammation of bronchioles or bronchopneumonia).

bronchus (bronchi).

(L. *bronchus,* air passage; Gr. *bronchos,* windpipe) bronch-; bronchi-; broncho-.

Ex: bronch-adenitis (inflammation of bronchial glands); bronchi-al (pertaining to a bronchus or a bronchium); bronchi-ectasis; bronch-itis (inflammation of bronchial tubes).

bud (germ; formative element; embryonic stage).

(Gr. *blastos,* bud) -blast-; blasto-.

Ex: blasto-derm (mass of cells produced by cleavage of a fertilized ovum); blasto-myces (genus of fungi). See also under *sprout.*

bursa (sac filled with fluid).

(L. *bursa,* pouch; Gr. *bursa,* wine skin) burs-; burso-.

Ex: burs-al (pertaining to a bursa); burs-ectomy (excision of a bursa); burs-itis (inflammation of a bursa); burso-lith (calculus in a bursa).

bursting. See under *break.*

buttock (rump).

(Gr. *pyge,* rump) -pyg-; pygo-.

Ex: pyg-algia (pain in a buttock); steato-pyg-ia (excessive deposit of fat on the buttocks); pygo-pagus (a double monster joined at the buttocks).

C

calcaneus. See under *heel bone.*

calcium (lime; chalk).

(L. *calx,* lime; *calcis*) calc-; calci-; calco-.

Ex: calc-emia (presence of too much calcium in the blood); calci-pexy (fixation of calcium in the tissues); calci-uria (presence of calcium in the urine); calco-spherite.

calculus. See under *stone.*

callus. See under *corn.*

cancer (carcinoma; malignancy).

(Gr. *karkinos,* crab) carcin-; carcino-.

Ex: carcin-ectomy (excision of a carcinoma); carcino-genic (producing cancer); carcino-phobia.

canthus (angle between eyelids).

(Gr. *kanthos,* canthus) canth-; cantho-.

Ex: canth-itis (inflammation of a canthus); cantho-plasty; cantho-rrhaphy (suture of a canthus).

capsule (box; case).

(L. *capsula,* box) capsul-; capsulo-.

Ex: capsul-ar (pertaining to a capsule); capsul-ation (formation of a capsule); capsul-ectomy (excision of a capsule); capsulo-rrhaphy (suture of a capsule); capsulo-tomy.

carbohydrate.

(L. *carbo,* coal; Gr. *hydor,* water) carbohydr-; carbohydrat-; carbohydro-.

Ex: carbohydr-ase (an enzyme which splits carbohydrates); carbohydrat-uria (presence of carbohydrates in the urine); carbohydro-genic (producing carbohydrates). See also *sugar.*

carbolic acid. See under *phenol.*

carbon (carbon dioxide).

(L. *carbo,* coal) carb-; carbo-; carbon-; carbono-.

Ex: carb-ide (compound of carbon and another substance); carbo-hydrate; carbon-ize (convert into coal); carbono-metry (measurement of carbon dioxide).

carbon dioxide. See under *carbon.*

carcinoma.

(Gr. *karkinoma,* cancer) carcin-; carcino-; carcinomat-; carcinomato-.

Ex: carcin-ectomy (excision of a carcinoma); carcino-genic (causing carcinoma or cancer); carcino-lysis (lysis of cancer cells); carcinomat-oid (resembling carcinoma); carcinomat-osis (presence of carcinomas); carcinomato-phobia (abnormal fear of cancer).

carcinoma. See under *cancer.*

cardiac sphincter. See under *heart.*

cardiac ventricle. See under *ventricle.*

carry (bring; convey; conduct).

(L. *ferre,* to bear) -fer; -fer-; -ferr-; -ferous.

Ex: a-ferr-ent (carrying toward a structure); e-ferr-ent (carrying away); sangui-ferous (carrying blood); urini-ferous (carrying urine); semini-ferous (carrying semen).

cartilage (gristle).

(Gr. *chondros,* cartilage) chondr-; chondro-.

Ex: chondr-ectomy (surgical excision of cartilage); chondro-dystrophy (abnormal development of cartilage); chondro-genic (forming cartilage).

case. See under *sheath.*

cation. See under *ion.*

causing. See under *inducing.*

cavity (hollow space).

(L. *cavitas,* hollow) cava-; cavi-; cavo-; cavit-.

Ex: cava-scope (an instrument used for examining cavities); cavit-ation (the formation of cavities); cavi-form (resembling a cavity); cavo-genic (causing the formation of cavities).

cavity, small. See under *alveolus.*

cell (compartment; chamber; enclosure).

(L. *cella,* cell, compartment; *cellula,* small cell) cell-; celli-; cello-; cellu-; cellul-; celluli-; cellulo-.

Ex: cell-ase (a kind of enzyme); celli-colous (living within cells); celli-form (like a cell); cello-biose (a sugar derived from cellulose); cellu-genic (producing cells); cellul-ar (pertaining to or composed of cells); cellul-itis (inflammation of cellular tissue); celluli-cidal (destructive to cells); cellulo-neuritis (inflammation of nerve cells).

cell (container; vessel; cover).

(Gr. kytos, hollow vessel) cyt-; -cyti-; cyto-.

Ex: cyt-ase (enzyme acting on cell wall); erythro-cyte; cytolytic (causing lysis of cells); cyto-plasm (protoplasm of a cell).

center (middle point; collection of nerve cells).

(Gr. *kentron;* L. *centrum,* center) centr-; centri-; centro-.

Ex: centr-ad (toward a center); centri-fugal (moving away from a center); centro-kinesia (movement caused by central stimulation).

cerebellum.

(L. *cerebellum,* little brain) cerebell-; cerebelli-; cerebello-.

Ex: cerebell-ar (pertaining to the cerebellum); cerebelli-fugal (moving away from the cerebellum); cerebello-pontine (pertaining to the cerebellum and the pons).

cerebral ventricle. See under *ventricle.*

cerebrum (brain).

(L. *cerebrum,* main portion of brain) cerebr-; cerebri-; cerebro-.

Ex: cerebr-al (pertaining to the cerebrum); cerebr-itis (inflammation of the brain); cerebri-form (shaped like the brain); cerebro-spinal (pertaining to the brain and the spinal cord).

cervix. See under *neck.*

chalk. See under *calcium.*

chamber. See under *cell.*

change. See under *development, mutation,* and *turn.*

changed (altered; transposed).

(Gr. *meta,* after, beyond) met-; meta-.

Ex: meta-bolism (the processes of change by which living substances are produced and broken down); meta-morphosis (change from one developmental stage to another); meta-stasis (the transfer or transposition of a pathologic condition from one place to another).

changing. See under *turning.*

characterized by (of the nature of; like).

(L. *-aceus*) -aceous.

Ex: membran-aceous (of the nature of a membrane); crust-aceous (characterized by the presence of a shell; having a crust).

chastisement. See under *punishment.*

checking. See under *stoppage.*

cheek (side of face).

(L. *bucca,* cheek) bucc-; bucco-.

Ex: bucc-al (pertaining to the cheek); bucco-lingual (pertaining to the cheek and tongue).

chemical action. See under *chemistry.*

chemistry (chemical substance; chemical action).

(Gr. *chemeia,* chemistry) chem-; chemi-; chemo-; chemico-.

Ex: chemico-cautery (cautery by means of a caustic chemical substance); chemo-taxis (movement of an organism in response to the influence of a chemical substance); chemo-therapy (treatment by means of chemical substances).

chest.

(Gr. *stethos,* chest) steth-; stetho-.

Ex: steth-algia (pain in the chest); stetho-graph (an instrument used to record the movements of the chest); stetho-scope; stetho-spasm (a spasm of the muscles of the chest).

chest (thorax).

(Gr. *thorax,* chest; genit. *thorakos*) thorac-; thoracico-; thoraco-.

Ex: thorac-algia (pain in the thorax); thoracico-humeral (pertaining to the chest and the humerus); thoraco-centesis (puncture of the chest wall); thoraco-lysis (the surgical freeing of the chest wall from adhesions).

chew (grind; masticate).

(Gr. *maseter,* a chewer) mas-; -mas-; masseter-; massetero-.

Ex: mas-esis (process of chewing); dys-masesis (difficult chewing); masseter-odynia (painful chewing); massetero-genous (caused by chewing).

chickenpox.

(L. *varicella*, chickenpox) varicell-; varicelli-.

Ex: varicell-ation (inoculation with varicella virus); varicelli-form (resembling chickenpox); varicelli-genous (caused by chickenpox).

child (infant).

(Gr. *pais*, child; genit. *paidos*) -ped-; pedo-.

Ex: ped-iatrics (branch of medicine dealing with children and children's diseases); ortho-ped-ics; pedo-phobia (fear of children).

childbirth (labor).

(Gr. *tokos*, childbirth) toco-; toko-; -toc-.

Ex: toco-ergometry (the measurement of the power of the uterine contractions during childbirth); toco-logy (the study of childbirth); toco-phobia (fear of childbirth); toko-dynamo-meter (a device for measuring the force of the uterine contractions during childbirth); dys-toc-ia (difficult labor).

childbirth (labor; parturition).

(L. *parturire*, be in labor) parturi-; parturio-; parturo-.

Ex: parturi-ent (designating a woman in labor); parturi-facient (a medicinal substance which initiates or facilitates labor); parturio-meter (an apparatus used to measure the expulsive power of the uterus).

childbirth, period following.

(L. *puerperium*, period following childbirth) puerper-; puerperal-.

Ex: puerper-a (a woman who has just given birth); puerperal-ism (any disorder resulting from childbirth); puerper-ium (the period immediately following childbirth or labor).

chin (lower jaw).

(Gr. *geneion*, chin; *genys*, lower jaw) geni-; genio-; geny-; genyo-.

Ex: micro-geni-a (smallness of the chin); genio-plasty (a plas-

tic operation on the chin); geny-cheiloplasty (a plastic operation on the lower jaw and the lip).

chin (lower jaw).

(L. *mentum,* chin) ment-; mento-.

Ex: ment-algia (pain in the chin); mento-labial (pertaining to
the chin and a lip).

choroid (chorion; envelope).

(Gr. *chorion,* membrane surrounding the fetus) chori-; chorio-;
choroid-; choroido-.

Ex: chorio-adenoma (an adenoma of the chorion); chorio-
amnionitis (inflammation of the chorion and amnion); chorio-
capillaris (the capillary layer of the choroid coat of the eyeball);
chorio-cele (herniation of the choroid coat of the eyeball);
chorio-genesis (development of the chorion of the fetus); cho-
rio-meningitis (inflammation of the choroid plexuses and the
meninges); chorion; chorion-itis (inflammation of the chorion;
also, inflammation of the corium); choroid-al (pertaining to
the choroid); choroido-retinitis (inflammation of the choroid
and the retina).

choroid plexus. See under *choroid.*

chromosomes, multiple of

(Gr. *-ploos,* -fold; *eidos,* form) -ploid.

Ex: ha-ploid (having a single set of chromosomes); di-ploid
(having two sets of chromosomes); poly-ploid (having several
sets of chromosomes).

chyle (juice).

(Gr. *chylos,* juice) chyl-; chyle-; chyli-; chylo-.

Ex: chyl-emia (presence of chyle in the blood); chyle-faction
(formation of chyle); chylo-rrhea (discharge of chyle).

cicatrix. See under *scar.*

ciliary body (circle).

(Gr. *kyklos,* circle) cycl-; cyclo-.

Ex: cycl-ectomy (excision of a portion of the ciliary body);
cycl-itis (inflammation of the ciliary body); cyclo-plegia (paralysis of the ciliary body).

circle (ring; round; rotation; gyrus).

(Gr. *gyros,* circle) -gyr-; gyro-.

Ex: gyr-ation (a rotatory movement); gyr-al (pertaining to a gyrus of the brain); oculo-gyr-ic (pertaining to the rotation of the eyeball); dextro-gyr-ation (a turning to the right or clockwise).

circle (rotation; round)

(Gr. *kyklos*, circle) cycl-; cycli-; cyclo-.

Ex: cycl-arthrosis (a joint permitting rotation); cycl-ic (occurring in cycles); cyclo-tropia; cyclo-phoria (a turning of the eyeball).

circle. See under *ciliary body.*

clan. See under *tribe.*

clavicle (collarbone; key).

(Gr. *kleis*, clavicle) cleid-; cleido-.

Ex: cleid-agra (pain in the clavicle); cleido-tomy (surgical cutting of the clavicle); sterno-cleido-mastoid (pertaining to the sternum, clavicle, and mastoid process).

claw. See under *nail.*

cleavage. See under *division.*

cleft (fissure; split).

(Gr. *schistos*, split) schist-; schisto-.

Ex: schist-asis (a splitting); schisto-cormia (a cleft condition of the trunk); schisto-glossia (a cleft condition of the tongue); schisto-thorax (a fissure of the chest).

close to. See under *near.*

closest. See under *nearest.*

clot. See under *embolus* and *thrombus.*

coccus (cocci; spherical microorganism).

(L. *coccus*, kernel) cocc-; cocci-; cocco-.

Ex: cocc-al (pertaining to cocci); cocco-genous (caused by cocci).

coccyx (coccygeal region).

(Gr. *kokkyx*, cuckoo, in allusion to its bill) coccy-; coccyg-; coccygo-.

Ex: coccy-algia (pain in the coccyx); coccyg-ectomy (surgical excision of the coccyx).

cold (low temperature).

(Gr. *psychros*, cold) psychro-.

Ex: psychro-esthesia (a condition in which a part of the body feels cold although it is warm); psychro-philic (thriving in low temperatures).

cold (frost; freezing).

(Gr. *kryos,* cold) cry-; cryo-.

Ex: cry-algesia (pain due to cold); cryo-cautery (cautery by means of extreme cold); cryo-gen (a substance producing cold).

collarbone. See under *clavicle.*

colon (large intestine).

(Gr. *kolon,* colon) col-; coli-; colo-; colon-.

Ex: col-itis (inflammation of the colon); colo-enteritis (inflammation of the colon and the small intestine); colon-ic (pertaining to the colon).

color (coloration; pigment; tint; hue).

(Gr. *chroma,* color; genit. *chromatos*) chrom-; chroma-; chromo-; chromato-.

Ex: chrom-affin (staining readily with chromium dyes); chroma-phil (staining readily); chromat-ic (pertaining to col- (or); chromato-plasm (the colored protoplasm of a pigmented cell).

compact. See under *thick.*

compartment. See under *cell.*

completely. See under *through.*

concave. See under *hollow.*

concealed. See under *hidden.*

concept. See under *idea.*

concretion. See under *stone.*

condition (habit).

(Gr. *hexis,* condition) -hex-; -hexi-; -hexis.

Ex: cac-hex-ia (condition of ill health); hexi-clastic (helping to break a habit); hexi-philia (proneness to acquire a habit); hexi-o-logy (the study of habits).

conduct. See under *carry* and *lead.*

conduction. See under *running.*

condyle (rounded projection; knuckle).

(Gr. *kondylos,* knuckle) condyl-; condylo-.

Ex: condyl-ar (pertaining to a condyle); condyl-ectomy (excision of a condyle); condylo-tomy (surgical incision into a condyle).

configuration. See under *form.*

conforming to rule. See under *normal.*

congenital absence.

(Gr.*ektrosis,* miscarriage) ect-; ectro-.

Ex: ectro-dactyly (congenital absence of a finger or toe); ectro-geny (congenital absence of an organ or structure); ectro-met-atarsia (congenital absence of a metatarsal bone).

connecting structure. See under *isthmus* and *yoke.*

consolidation. See under *immobility.*

contact. See under *touch.*

contracted. See under *narrow.*

contrary. See under *against.*

contrary to. See under *opposite.*

convey. See under *carry.*

cord (string; tract; fold).

(Gr. *chorde,* cord) chord-; chordo-.

Ex: chord-itis (inflammation of a cord, as the spermatic cord); chordo-tomy (surgical cutting of a nerve tract).

corium of skin. See under *choroid.*

corn (callus).

(Gr. *helos,* nail) hel-; hela-; helo.

Ex: hel-ectomy (excision of a corn or callus); hela-clinia (tendency to develop corns or calluses); hel-odynia (pain caused by a corn or callus); hel-osis (the presence of corns or calluses); helo-tomy (the surgical cutting of a corn or callus).

cornea of eye.

(Gr. *keras,* cornea; genit. *keratos*) kerat-; kerati-; kerato-.

Ex: kerat-algia (pain in the cornea); kerat-itis (inflammation of the cornea); kerato-centesis (surgical puncture of the cornea).

corpse. See under *death.*

corpus luteum (lutein).

(L. *luteus,* yellow) lute-; lutein-.

Ex: lute-al (pertaining to the corpus luteum); lute-ectomy (excision of a corpus luteum); lutein-ization.

correct. See under *normal.*

cortex (rind; outer layer; bark).

(L. *cortex,* bark; genit. *corticis*) corti-; cortic-; cortici-; cortico-.
Ex: corti-adrenal (pertaining to the cortex of the adrenal gland); cortici-fugal (moving away from the cortex); cortico-tropic (influencing the cortex).

countenance. See under *face.*

cranium (skull).

(L. *cranium,* skull; Gr. *kranion*) crani-; cranio-.
Ex: crani-ectomy (excision of a part of the cranium); cranio-clast (an instrument for crushing the fetal skull); cranio-logy (the study of skulls).

craving. See under *mania.*

crescent. See under *sickle.*

crest (ridge; tuft).

(Gr. *lophos,* ridge) loph-; lophi-; lophio-; lopho-.
Ex: lophio-stomate (having a crested structure or stoma); lopho-dont (having ridged molars); lopho-trichous (having a tuft of flagella).

cricoid cartilage.

(Gr. *krikos,* ring) cric-; crico-; cricoid-.
Ex: crico-arytenoid (pertaining to the cricoid cartilage and arytenoid cartilage); cricoid-ectomy (excision of the cricoid cartilage); crico-thyroid (pertaining to the cricoid and thyroid cartilages).

crooked. See under *bent* and *curved.*

crystalline lens. See under *lens.*

current. See under *flow.*

curve. See under *bend.*

curved (crooked; twisted).

(Gr. *skolios,* crooked) scolio-; scolioso-; scoliot-.
Ex: scolio-kyphosis (a deformity consisting of scoliosis and kyphosis); scolioso-meter (a device for measuring curves); scoliot-ic (affected by scoliosis). See also *twisted.*

custom. See under *law.*

cut. See under *incision.*

cutis. See under *skin.*

cutting (surgical incision).

(Gr. *tome,* a cutting) -tom-; -tome; tomo-; -tomy.
Ex: micro-tome (an instrument for cutting thin layers of tissue); tomo-mania (an abnormal desire to undergo surgery); thoraco-tomy (a surgical incision into the chest). See also *section.*

cylinder (column; roller).

(Gr. *kylindros,* roller) cylindr-; cylindri-; cylindro-.
Ex: cylindr-arthrosis (a joint with cylindrical articular surfaces); cylindri-form (shaped like a cylinder); cylindro-cellular (composed of cylindrical cells).

cyst.

(Gr. *kystis,* sac) -cyst-; cysti-; cystido-; cysto-.
Ex: poly-cyst-ic (containing many cysts); cyst-oma (a tumor containing neoplastic cysts); cysti-cercus (a form of larval tapeworm situated in a cyst-like structure); cystido-genic (producing cysts); cysto-adenoma (an adenoma containing cysts). See also *bladder.*

cyst of ovary.

(Gr. *oophoron,* ovary; *kystis,* sac) oophorocyst-; oophorocysto-.
Ex: oophorocyst-ectomy (excision of an ovarian cyst); oophorocysto-tomy (a cutting into an ovarian cyst); oophorocyst-osis (the presence or formation of ovarian cysts).

D

dampness. See under *moisture.*
dark spot. See under *darkness.*
darkness (dark spot).

(Gr. *skotos,* darkness) scoto-.
Ex: scoto-meter (an instrument for locating and measuring scotomas); scoto-philia (a preference for darkness); scoto-phobia; scot-opia (vision in semidarkness).

darkness. See under *night.*
dead. See under *decaying.*
dead tissue. See under *death.*
dearth. See under *deficiency.*

death.

(Gr. *thanatos,* death) thanat-; thanato-.

Ex: thanati-form (resembling death); thanato-logy (the study of death); thanat-ophidia (deadly snakes or serpents); thanato-phobia (abnormal fear of death).

death (dead; dead tissue; corpse).

(Gr. *nekros,* dead body) necr-; necrot-; necroto-; necro-.

Ex: necr-ectomy (excision of dead tissue); necro-philism (sexual interest in a corpse); necro-coitus (coitus with a corpse); necro-phobia (excessive fear of death); necroto-logy (the study of death and the changes produced by death).

death (dying).

(L. *mors,* death; genit; *mortis*) mort-; morti-.

Ex: mort-al; mort-ician (person trained in preparing the dead for burial); morti-natality (ratio of stillbirths to the general birth rate); morti-ferous (capable of causing death).

decay (decomposition; rot).

(Gr. *pythein,* to rot) pyth-; pytho-.

Ex: pytho-genic (promoting decay; causing decomposition); pytho-genous (caused by decay); pytho-philic (thriving in filth).

decaying (putrefying; dead).

(Gr. *sapros,* rotten) sapr-; sapro-.

Ex: sapr-emia (the presence in the blood of decaying matter); sapro-genic (causing decay); sapro-phyte (a microorganism living on decaying matter); sapro-zoic (living on dead matter).

deceptive. See under *false.*

decomposition. See under *decay* and *putrefaction.*

decrease. See under *less.*

defense. See under *protection.*

deficiency (scarcity; dearth; poverty).

(Gr. *penia,* scarcity) -penia-.

Ex: erythro-penia (a deficiency of red blood cells); thrombo-penia (a deficiency of thrombin); kineto-penia (dearth of movement or activity); phreno-penia (poverty of emotional response); eroto-penia (subnormal sexual desire).

deficiency. See under *stoppage.*

deficient. See under *few.*

deformed. See under *maimed.*

deglutition. See under *swallowing.*

deity. See under *god.*

delicate. See under *slender.*

dense. See under *thick.*

depict. See under *paint.*

derivation from. See under *from.*

derma. See under *skin.*

descent. See under *birth.*

describe. See under *write.*

desire. See under *appetite.*

destruction. See under *dissolution.*

development (change; growth).

(Gr. *plassein,* to mold; *plasis,* a molding) -plasia; -plasis.
Ex: hyper-plasia (excessive development); hypo-plasia; meta-plasia (the develement of a particular tissue from cells which normally develop another type of tissue); macro-plasia (over-growth of a part).

diaphragm (phrenic nerve).

(Gr. *phren,* diaphragm) -phren-; phrenic-; phrenico-; phreno-.
Ex: sub-phren-ic (situated under the diaphragm); phrenic-ectomy (excision of a part of the phrenic nerve); phrenico-tomy (the surgical cutting of the phrenic nerve); phreno-hepat-ic (pertaining to the diaphragm and the liver).

different. See under *other.*

difficult (laborious; unsuccessful).

(Gr. *mogis,* with difficulty) mogi-.
Ex: mogi-graphia (condition marked by difficulty in writing); mogi-lalia (difficulty in speaking); mogi-tocia (difficult child-birth).

difficult (painful; hard; faulty; impaired; unlike).

(Gr.) dys-.
Ex: dys-adrenia (impaired function of the adrenal glands); dys-arthria (faulty articulation in speech); dys-entery (painful intestine); dys-kinesia (impairment of the power of move-ment); dys-ostosis (faulty ossification); dys-pepsia (impaired

digestion); dys-phagia (difficult swallowing); dys-pnea (difficulty of breathing); dys-trophy (faulty nutrition and development).

digestion (digest; digestive).
　(Gr. *peptein,* to digest) -peps-; pept-; pepto-.
　Ex: dys-peps-ia (impairment of digestion); eu-pept-ic (marked
　by good digestion); pepto-genic (stimulating digestion).

digit (finger; toe).
　(L. *digitus,* finger, toe) digit-; digiti-; digito-.
　Ex: digit-al (pertaining to a finger or toe); digiti-grade (walk-
　ing on the toes).

direction. See under *bearing.*

discharge. See under *flow.*

discharge, excessive. See under *flow, excessive.*

discipline. See under *punishment.*

discomfort. See under *pain.*

discourse. See under *word.*

disease (illness; disorder).
　(Gr. *nosos,* disease) nos-; noso-.
　Ex: noso-graphy (a description of diseases or a disease); noso-
　philia (an abnormal desire to be sick); noso-poietic (causing
　disease).

disease (illness; disorder).
　(Gr. *pathos,* disease) -path; -path-; patho-; -pathy; -pathia.
　Ex: psycho-path (a person affected by a psychosis); histo-
　patho-logy; patho-genic (causing disease); patho-gnomonic
　(indicative of a particular disease); toxico-pathy (a disease
　caused by a toxin); myo-pathia (a disease of a muscle).

disk (intervertebral disk).
　(Gr. *disks,* disk; L. *discus*) disco-; discoid-.
　Ex: disco-genic (caused by or originating in an intervertebral
　disk); discoid-ectomy (excision of an intervertebral disk); dis-
　co-pathy (disease of an intervertebral disk).

dislike. See under *hate.*

disorder. See under *disease.*

dissolution (dissolving; destruction; loosing).
　(Gr. *lysis,* a loosening) lys-; lysi-; -lysis; lyso-.

Ex: lys-emia (dissolution of blood cells); lysi-meter (an instrument to determine solubility); hemo-lysis (dissolution of red blood cells and the liberation of the hemoglobin); auto-lysis (dissolution of cells by their own enzymes).

dissolving. See under *solution.*

distal (farther; remote; farther from median line).

(L. *distantia,* distance) dist-; disto-.

Ex: disto-buccal (pertaining to the distal and buccal surfaces of a tooth); disto-lingual (pertaining to the distal and lingual surfaces of a tooth).

distant. See under *far away.*

division (cleavage).

(Gr. *schizein,* to divide) schiz-; schizo-.

Ex: schiz-axon (a divided axon); schizo-genesis (reproduction by division or fission); schizo-phrenia; schizo-trichia (splitting of the hairs).

dizziness. See under *vertigo.*

dog (canine; bark).

(Gr. *kyon,* dog) cyn-; cyni-; cyno-.

Ex: cyn-anthropy (insanity in which the patient believes he is a dog); cyn-iatrics (branch of veterinary medicine dealing with dogs); cyno-phobia (abnormal fear of dogs).

dormant. See under *sleep.*

dorsum. See under *back.*

dose (dosage).

(Gr. *dosis,* dose) dos-; dosi-; doso-.

Ex: dos-age (administration of medicines in regulated doses); micro-dos-age (administration of minute doses); dosi-metry (the scientific determination of doses); doso-genic (determining or influencing the dose).

dot. See under *point.*

double (twice; twofold; twin).

(Gr. *diploos,* double) diplo-.

Ex: diplo-bacillus (a bacillus occurring in pairs); diplo-coria (double pupil); diplo-pia (double vision); diplo-neural (having a double innervation). See also *both* and *two.*

down (downward).

    (Gr. *kata,* down) kat-; kata-.

    Ex: kata-basis (a downward slipping of a structure); kata-sexual (having a sexual interest in lower animals); kata-phrenia (a downward trend of the mood).

down (low; inferior; under; along with).

    (Gr. *kata,* down) cata-.

    Ex: cata-basis (decline of a disease); cata-bolism (process of breaking down); cata-rrh (discharge of mucus); cata-stalsis (a downward moving wave of contraction).

downward displacement. See under *drooping.*

dream (night dreams).

    (Gr. *oneiros,* dream) oneir-; oneiro-.

    Ex: oneiro-analysis (analysis of dreams); oneir-odynia (distress caused by a nightmare); oneiro-clinic (having a tendency to dream).

driving away (moving away; fleeing; ephemeral).

    (L. *fugere,* flee) -fug-; -fugal; -fuge.

    Ex: centri-fugal (moving away from the center); vermi-fuge (something that expels worms).

drooping (downward displacement; sagging; falling).

    (Gr. *ptosis,* a falling) -ptosis.

    Ex: viscero-ptosis (a downward displacement of the viscera); blepharo-ptosis (a drooping of the eyelid); gastro-ptosis (a sagging of the stomach); entero-ptosis (a downward displacement of the intestine).

drug (medicinal substance).

    (Gr. *pharmakon,* drug) pharmac-; pharmaceut-; pharmaco-.

    Ex: pharmac-al (pertaining to pharmacy or drugs); pharmaceut-ical; pharmaco-dynamics (the study of the action of drugs or medicinal substances); pharmaco-peia (an official book on drugs); pharmaco-therapy (the treatment of disease with medicinal substances).

dryness.

    (Gr. *xeros,* dry) xero-.

    Ex: xero-cheilia (dryness of the lips); xero-derma (dryness of the skin); xero-mycteria (dryness of the mucous membrane of the nose); xero-stomia (dryness of the mouth).

ductus deferens. See under *vessel.*

dung. See under *feces* and *excrement.*

duodenum.

(L. *duodenum digitorum,* of twelve fingers' breath) duoden-; duodeno-.

Ex: duoden-itis (inflammation of the duodenum); duodeno-cystostomy (formation of an anastomosis between the duodenum and the gallbladder); duodeno-hepatic (pertaining to the duodenum and the liver).

durable. See under *long.*

duration. See under *time.*

dwarfishness. See under *smallness*

E

ear.

(Gr. *ous,* ear; genit. *otos*) -ot-; oto-.

Ex: ot-algia (pain in an ear); peri-ot-ic (surrounding an ear); par-ot-id (situated near or beside the ear); ot-itis (inflammation of an ear); oto-logy (branch of medicine dealing with the ear); oto-mycosis (infection of the ear by a fungus).

ear (hearing).

(L. *auris,* ear) auricul-; auriculo-.

Ex: auricul-ar (pertaining to the ear); sub-auricular (below the ear); auriculo-cranial (pertaining to the ear and the cranium).

eardrum (membrana tympani).

(L. *myringa,* membrane) myring-; myringo-.

Ex: myring-ectomy (excision of the eardrum); myring-itis (inflammation of the eardrum); myringo-mycosis (a fungus infection of the eardrum).

earlier. See under *before.*

earliest (first; original; primitive).

(Gr. *protos,* first) prot-; proto-.

Ex: prot-anopia (a type of defect in color vision); proto-neuron (the first neuron in a reflex arc); proto-plasm; proto-spasm (the earliest of a series of spasms).

early. See under *old.*

earth (soil; dirt).

(Gr. *ge,* earth) geo-.

Ex: geo-phagia (the eating of soil or turf); geo-medicine (medicine dealing with the effect of the geographical environment on health); geo-tropism (tropism exerted by the gravity of the earth).

earthworm (roundworm; worm).

(L. *lumbricus,* earthworm) lumbri-; lumbric-.

Ex: lumbri-cide (an agent which destroys earthworms and similar worms); lumbric-oid (like an earthworm); lumbric-osis (infestation with worms).

easily. See under *good.*

eating (ingestion; engulfing).

(Gr. *phagein,* to eat) -phag-; phagia; -phagy-; phago-.

Ex: mono-phag-ism (subsistence on one kind of food); omo-phagia (the eating of uncooked food); scato-phagy (the eating of excrement or feces); phago-cytosis (the engulfing of micro-organisms, etc); phago-phobia (fear of eating). See also *food.*

edge. See under *lip.*

egg (ovum; female reproductive cell).

(Gr. *oon,* an egg) oo-.

Ex: oo-genesis (the development of an ovum); oo-gonium (the early cell from which an ovum develops); oo-sperm (a fertilized ovum in the early stages). See also *ovum.*

eight (eight times).

(Gr. *okto,* eight) oct-; octa-; octo-; octi-.

Ex: oct-ane (a hydrocarbon having eight carbon atoms); octo-valent (having a chemical valence of eight); octi-para (a woman who has borne eight children in eight pregnancies); octo-genarian (a person who is between 80 and 89 years old).

elaboration. See under *secretion.*

elastic (resilient; springy).

(Gr. *elastikos,* elastic) elast-; elasti-; elasto-.

Ex: elast-ase (enzyme digesting elastic tissue); elasto-fibroma (a tumor composed of elastic and fibrous tissue); elasto-lytic (dissolving elastic tissue).

elbow joint (elbow).

(Gr. *olene,* elbow; *kranion,* head; *arthron,* joint) olecranarthr-; olecranarthro-.

Ex: olecranarthr-itis (arthritis of the elbow); olecranarthro-pathy (any disease of the elbow joint).

elderly. See under *old age.*

electric current. See under *flow.*

electricity.

(Gr. *elektron,* amber) electr-; electri-; electro-.

Ex: electr-ic (pertaining to electricity); electri-fy; electro-cardio-gram; electro-kinetic (pertaining to motion produced by elec-tricity).

elevation. See under *height.*

elongated. See under *long.*

embolus (plug; clot).

Gr. *embolos,* plug) embol-; emboli-; embolo-.

Ex: embol-ectomy (excision of an embolus); emboli-form (re-sembling an embolus); embolo-genic (producing an embolus); embolo-lytic (dissolving an embolus).

embryo.

(Gr. *embryon,* embryo) embry-; embryo-.

Ex: embry-ectomy (excision of an embryo); embryo-genesis (the development of an embryo); embryo-logy (the science of embryos).

emotion. See under *mind.*

encephalon. See under *brain.*

encircling. See under *around.*

end (termination).

(Gr. *telos,* end) tel-; tele-; telo-.

Ex: tel-angiectasis (dilatation of capillaries or end vessels); tele-neuron (a nerve ending); telo-dendron (a terminal branch of an axon); telo-phase (the end phase of mitosis). See also *limb.*

energy. See under *work.*

engulfing. See under *eating.*

enlarged. See under *large.*

entire (whole; exclusively).

(Gr. *holos,* entire) hol-; holo-.

Ex: hol-andric (transmitted exclusively through the male line); holo-blastic (designating a cleavage in which the entire ovum takes part); holo-gynic (transmitted exclusively through the female line); holo-systolic (involving the entire systole).

enzyme.

(Gr. *zyme,* ferment) zymo-.

Ex: xymo-gen (the precursor of an enzyme); zymo-lysis (lysis by an enzyme or ferment); zymo-phore (the active group of an enzyme molecule).

equal (of same quantity, intensity, etc.).

(L. *aequus,* equal) equa-; equi-.

Ex: equi-potential (having equal power); equi-lateral (having equal sides); equi-molecular (having an equal number of molecules).

equal (same; identical; similar; alike).

(Gr. *isos,* equal) is-; iso-.

Ex: is-auxesis (equal growth of a part and the whole); iso-caloric (containing the same number of calories); iso-metropia (condition of having the same power of refraction in both eyes); iso-thermic (having the same temperature).

erected. See under *straight.*

esophagus (gullet).

(L. *oesophagus,* esophagus) esophag-; esophago-.

Ex: esophag-ectasia (dilatation of the esophagus); esophag-itis; esophago-cele (herniation of the esophagus); esophago-plasty (plastic surgery on the esophagus).

estrus (sexual urge).

(Gr. *oistros,* keen desire) estra-; estri-; estro-.

Ex: estri-nization (production of the cellular changes); estro-genic (producing estrus).

even (level; smooth; equilibrium).

(Gr. *homalos,* even) homal-; homali-; homalo-.

Ex: homal-onychous (having smooth nails); homali-thermia (evenness of the body temperature); homalo-phrenia (evenness of temper); homalo-sphygmia (smoothness of the pulse); homalo-trophic (supplying the proper level of nutrition).

every. See under *all.*

everywhere. See under *all.*

examining. See under *viewing.*

excess. See under *more.*

excessive (more than normal; above; over).

(Gr. *hyper,* above) hyper-.

Ex: hyper-acidity (excessive acidity); hyper-calcemia (excess of calcium in the blood); hyper-esthesia (increased sensitivity, as of the skin); hyper-ostosis (overgrowth of bone).

excessive. See under *above, beyond,* and *many.*

excision.

(Gr. *ek,* out; *temnein,* to cut) -ectomize; -ectomy.

Ex: nephr-ectomize (to excise or remove a kidney); adrenal-ectomize (to excise the adrenal glands); append-ectomy; ton-sill-ectomy.

excite (urge; set in motion; spur).

(Gr. *hormaein,* excite) horm-; hormon-; hormono-.

Ex: horm-ary (exciting); hormon-e; hormon-al; hormon-ago-gue (a substance which stimulates the secretion of a hormone); hormono-therapy (treatment involving the use of hormones).

exciting. See under *stimulating.*

exclusively. See under *entire.*

excrement (dung; fecal matter).

(Gr. *skor,* excrement; genit. *skatos*) scat-; scato-.

Ex: scat-acratia (inability to control the feces); scato-logy (the study of feces); scato-phagy (the perversion of eating feces); scato-philia (an abnormal interest in fecal matter).

exertion. See under *work.*

existence (being).

(Gr. *on,* a being; genit. *ontos*) onto-.

Ex: onto-genesis (the development of an individual organism); onto-logy (the science of being); onto-cycle (a biological cycle in which an old organism assumes the characteristic of a young organism).

exposed. See under *naked.*

external. See under *outside.*

extremity. See under *limb.*

eye (eyeball).

(L. *oculus,* eye) ocul-; oculi-; oculo-.

Ex: ocul-ar (pertaining to the eye); oculi-form (shaped like an eye); oculo-motor (pertaining to the movements of the eyeball); oculo-pathy (any disease of the eye).

eye (eyeball; ophthalmos).

(Gr. *ophthalmos,* eye) ophthalm-; ophthalmo-.

Ex: ophthalm-itis (inflammation of an eye); ophthalmo-meter (an instrument for measuring the refractive power of the eye); ophthalmo-plegia (paralysis of the muscles of the eye).

eye. See under *optics* and *vision.*

eye socket. See under *orbit.*

eyelash (eyelid; hair-like process; ciliary process).

(L. *cilium,* eyelash) cil-; cili-; cilio-.

Ex: cili-ary (pertaining to eyelashes, eyelids, cilia, the ciliary body, etc.); cili-ectomy (excision of a portion of the ciliary body); cilio-scleral (pertaining to the ciliary process and the sclera); super-cili-um (structure above the eyelid, i.e., the eyebrow).

eyelid. (Gr. *blepharon,* eyelid) blephar-; blepharo-.

Ex: blephar-ism (spasm of an eyelid); blephar-itis (inflammation of an eyelid); blepharo-ptosis (drooping of an eyelid); blepharo-tomy (an incision of an eyelid).

eyelid (palpebra).

(L. *palpebra,* eyelid) -palpebr-.

Ex: palpebr-al (pertaining to the eyelids); palpebr-ate (to move the eyelids); inter-palpebral (between the eyelids); infra-palpebral (below the eyelid).

F

face (aspect; appearance).

(L. *facies,* face) faci-; facio-.

Ex: facio-cervical (pertaining to the face and neck); facio-plasty (a plastic operation on the face); cranio-faci-al (pertaining to the cranium and the face); faci-odynia (pain in the face).

face (countenance).

(Gr. *prosopon,* face) prosop-; prosopo-.

Ex: prosop-agnosia (inability to recognize faces); prosopo-neuralgia (neuralgia of the face); prosopo-scopy (examination of the face).

facial expression. See under *nature.*

falling. See under *drooping.*

false (deceptive; illusory; spurious; pretended).

(Gr. *pseudein,* to deceive) pseud-; pseudo-.

Ex: pseud-arthritis (a disorder resembling arthritis; false arthritis); pseudo-cast (a false urinary cast); pseudo-chorea (a condition marked by symptoms deceptively similar to those of chorea); pseudo-edema (a puffiness resembling edema); pseudo-pregnancy (false pregnancy).

far away (distant).

(Gr. *tele,* far off) tel-; tele-.

Ex: tel-algia (pain in a part distant from the actual source of pain); tele-cardiography; tele-ceptor (a receptor of stimuli originating at a distance).

farther See under *distal.*

fascia (band of fibrous tissue).

(L. *fascia,* band) fasci-; fascio-.

Ex: extra-fasci-al (situated outside a fascia); fasci-itis (inflammation of a fascia); fascio-lysis (the loosening of a fascia); fascio-plasty (plastic surgery on a fascia).

fast. See under *rapid.*

fat (fatness; fatty tissue).

(Gr. *pimelo,* fat) pimel-; pimelo-.

Ex: pimel-oma (a tumor composed of fatty tissue); pimelogenic (producing fat); pimelo-pexis (fixation of fat); pimelo-phagia (the eating of food rich in fat).

fat (oil).

(Gr. *lipos,* fat) lip-; liparo-; lipo-.

Ex: lip-ase (an enzyme which decomposes fats); liparo-cele (a hernia containing a mass of fat); lipo-genic (producing fat).

fat (suet).

(L. *adeps,* fat; genit. *adipis*) adip-; adipo-.

Ex: adip-ectomy (excision of masses of fat); adipo-cele (a hernia in which the protruding mass is fat); adipo-genic (producing fat); adipo-lytic (causing the splitting of fat); adip-osis (an excessive deposit of fat in the body); adipo-pexia (fixation of fat).

fat (tallow).

(Gr. *stear,* fat; genit. *steatos*) stear-; stearo-; steat-; steato-.

Ex: stear-ate (a compound of stearic acid); stearo-dermia (a disorder of the sebaceous glands); steat-itis (inflammation of fatty tissue); steato-genic (producing fat).

father (male ancestor).

(L. *pater,* father; genit. *patris*) patri-; patro-.

Ex: patri-lineal (discended through the male ancestors); patro-clinous (inherited from the father); patro-latry (excessive devotion to one's father).

fatty secretion. See under *sebum.*

fatty tissue. See under *fat.*

faulty. See under *difficult* and *improper.*

fear (aversion for).

(Gr. *phobos,* fear) -phobia; phobo-.

Ex: patho-phobia (abnormal fear of illness); terato-phobia (fear of bearing a deformed child); iatro-phobia (fear of physicians); ophidio-phobia (fear of snakes); phobo-genic (inducing fear); phobo-phobia (fear of fear).

fecal matter. See under *feces* and *excrement.*

feces (dung; excrement; stool).

(Gr. *kopros,* dung) copr-; copro-.

Ex: copr-acrasia (inability to retain the feces); copro-lagnia (sexual excitation derived from sight of feces); copro-lith (fecal concretion).

feces (excrement; dung; dregs).

(L. *faex,* excrement; genit. *faecis;* pl. *faeces*) fec-; feca-; feci-; feco-.

Ex: fec-al (of the nature of feces); feca-lith (a concretion formed of fecal matter); feco-lagnia (sexual desire aroused by sight of feces).

feces (stool; dung).

(L. *stercus,* dung) sterco-; stercor-.

Ex: sterco-bilin (a pigment occurring in the feces); sterco-lith (a concretion formed from fecal matter); stercor-oma (a mass in the rectum composed of fecal matter); stercor-ous (fecal).

feel with hand. See under *touch.*

feeling. See under *sensation.*

female. See under *woman.*

female sex organs. See under *vulva.*

femur (thighbone).

(L. *femur,* thigh) femor-; femori-; femoro-.

Ex: tibio-femor-al (pertaining to the tibia and femur); femoro-iliac (pertaining to the femur and the ilium); retro-femoral (situated behind the femur).

fermentation.

(Gr. *zyme,* ferment) zymo-.

Ex: zymo-chemistry (the chemistry of fermentation); zymo-logy (the study of fermentation); zymo-phyte (a microorganism causing fermentation).

ferrous. See under *iron.*

fetal monster. See under *monster.*

fetus (newborn).

(L. *fetus,* offspring) fet-; feti-; feto-.

Ex: fet-ation (development of a fetus in the uterus); feti-cide (killing of a fetus); feto-placental (pertaining to a fetus and the placenta).

fever (heat).

(Gr. *pyr,* fire; *pyretos,* heat) pyr-; pyre-; pyret-; pyreto-; pyrex-; pyro-.

Ex: pyr-emia (presence of pyrogenic substances in the blood); pyre-therapy (treatment of disease by means of fever); pyret-ic (pertaining to fever); pyreto-gen (a substance which produces fever); pyrex-ia (fever); pyro-gen (a substance capable of producing fever).

fever (pyrexia).

(L. *febris,* fever) febri-; febro-; febr-.

Ex: febri-facient (inducing fever); febri-fuge (a substance which reduces fever); febr-ile (having fever).

few (little; deficient; insufficient; scanty).

(Gr. *oligos,* small) olig-; oligo-.

Ex: olig-emia (a deficiency of blood); olig-idria (insufficient perspiration); oligo-menorrhea (scanty menstruation); oligo-spermia (the presence of few spermatozoa in the semen).

fewness. See under *scarcity.*

fiber (thread-like structure).

(L. *fibra,* fiber) fibr-; fibra-; fibri-; fibro-.

Ex: fibr-oma (a tumor of fibrous tissue); fibro-plasia (growth of fibrous tissue). See also *fibril.*

fibril (tiny filament; minute fiber).

(L. *fibrilla,* small filament) fibrill-; fibrillo-.

Ex: fibrill-ar (pertaining to fibrillae or fibrils); fibrillo-genesis (formation of fibrils); fibrillo-lytic (disintegrating fibrils).

fibrin.

(Gr. *is,* fiber; genit. *inos*) inos-.

Ex: inos-emia (increase of fibrin in the blood); inos-uria (increase of amount of fibrin in the urine).

fibrin.

(L. *fibra,* fiber) fibrin-; fibrino-.

Ex: fibrin-emia (presence of excessive amount of fibrin in the blood); fibrino-gen (a protein forming fibrin); fibrino-lysin (an enzyme which aids the digestion of fibrin).

fibrous. See under *hard.*

fifth.

(L. *quintus,* fifth) quint-; quinti-; quintu-.

Ex: quint-an (recurring on the fifth day); quinti-gravida (a woman who is pregnant for the fifth time); quintu-plet (one of five infants born in one labor).

fibrous tissue (fiber; muscle).

(Gr. *is,* fiber; genit. *inos*) ino-; inos-.

Ex: ino-cyte (a cell of fibrous connective tissue); inos-itis (inflammation of fibrous tissue).

filament, small. See under *fibril.*

finger (toe; digit).

(Gr. *daktylos,* finger) dactyl-; dactyli-; dactylo-.

Ex: dactyl-edema (swelling of a finger or toe); dactyl-itis; dactylo-gryposis (permanent flexion of a finger or toe); dactylo-spasm. See also *digit.*

fingernail. See under *nail.*

firm. See under *hard.*

firm, making. See under *fixation.*

first. See under *earliest.*

first time (for the first time).

(L. *primus,* first) primi-.

Ex: primi-gravida (a woman pregnant for the first time); primi-para (a woman who is giving birth for the first time); primi-genial (formed first).

fish (fish-like).

(Gr. *ichthys,* fish) ichthy-; ichthyo-.

Ex. ichthy-ism (poisoning by a toxin found in fish); ichthy-osis (a disease marked by scaliness of the skin); ichthyo-toxin (a toxin occurring in fish).

fissure. See under *cleft.*

fistula (abnormal channel).

(L. *fistula,* pipe) fistul-; fistula-; fistuli-; fistulo-.

Ex: fistul-ectomy (excision of a fistula); fistuli-zation (the formation of a fistula); fistulo-tomy (a surgical cutting into a fistula).

fistula. See under *tube.*

five.

(Gr. *pente,* five) pent-; penta-; penti-; pento-.

Ex: penta-digital (having five digits); penta-valent (having a valence of five); penti-para (a woman who is bearing a child for the fifth time); pent-ose (a sugar having five carbon atoms); pento-gamous (pertaining to five marriages).

five.

(L. *quinque,* five) quinque-.

Ex: quinque-cuspid (a tooth having five cusps); quinque-tubercular (having five tubercles); quinque-valent (having a chemical valence of five); quinque-tocous (having five children).

fixation (attachment; securing; making firm).

(Gr. *pegnynai,* to fasten; *pexis,* a fixing; *pagos,* fixation) -pexy; -pagus.

Ex: nephro-pexy (fixation of a loose kidney); gastro-pexy (fixation of the stomach); hystero-pexy (fixation of the uterus); cranio-pagus (a double fetal monster in which the heads are united).

flagellum. See under *whip.*

flake. See under *scale.*

flank (loin; abdominal wall; abdomen).

(Gr. *lapara,* flank) lapar-; laparo-.

Ex: lapar-ectomy (surgical excision of a portion of the abdominal wall); laparo-cystectomy (excision of a cyst through an abdominal incision); laparo-scopy (inspection of the interior of the abdomen); laparo-tomy (a surgical incision into the abdominal wall, especially at the flank).

flat. See under *wide.*

flea.

(L. *pulex,* flea; genit. *pulicis*) pulic-; pulici-; pul-.

Ex: pulic-osis (the disorder caused by the bites of fleas); pulici-cide (an agent which kills fleas); de-pul-ization (the process of freeing from fleas).

fleeing. See under *driving away.*

flesh.

(Gr. *sarx,* flesh; genit. *sarkos*) sarc-; sarco-.

Ex: sarco-genic (forming flesh or muscle tissue); sarc-oid (resembling flesh); sarco-lemma (the sheath surrounding a striated muscle fiber); sarc-oma; sarco-plasm (the matter surrounding the fibrillae of a muscle fiber).

flex. See under *bend.*

flow (current; electric current).

(Gr. *rheos,* current) rheo-.

Ex: rheo-meter (an instrument for measuring the blood current); rheo-stat (an instrument for controlling an electric current); rheo-taxis (orientation parallel with the direction of a current).

flow (discharge).

(Gr. *rhein,* to flow)-rrhea.

Ex: meno-rrhea (normal menstrual flow); dia-rrhea; leuko-rrhea (a whitish discharge from the vagina); gono-rrhea; oto-rrhea (a discharge from the ear).

flow, excessive (excessive discharge).

(Gr. *rhegnynai,* to burst) -rrhage; -rrhagia.

Ex: balano-rrhagia (a copious discharge from the glans penis); bleno-rrhagia (a discharge of mucus); gastro-rrhagia (a hemorrhage from the stomach); meno-rrhagia (excessive menstrual discharge); hemo-rrhage; lympho-rrhagia (a discharge of lymph).

fluctuate. See under *oscillate.*

fluid. See under *liquid, moisture,* and *water.*

fold (ridge).

(L. *plicare,* to fold) -plic-; plica-; plici-; plicato-.

Ex: du-plic-ation (a folding in two); plic-ation (an operation in which a muscle is shortened by the formation of tucks or folds); plici-ferous (having folds); plicato-undulate (folded and wavy).

follicle (small sac; gland).

(L. *folliculus,* small bag) follicul-.

Ex: follicul-ar (pertaining to a follicle); follicul-itis (inflammation of a follicle); follicul-osis (presence of excessive number of lymph follicles).

following. See under *after.*

food (eating).

(Gr. *sitos,* food) sito-.

Ex: sito-logy (the study of food and eating habits); sito-phobia (fear of eating); sito-therapy (diet therapy).

food (nourishment).

(L. *cibus,* food) cib-; ciba-; cibo-.

Ex: ciba-rious (edible); cibo-phobia (fear of food); cibo-genous (caused by food).

food. See under *nutrition.*

foot (foot-like structure).

(L. *pes,* foot; genit. *pedis*) ped-; pedi-; pedo-.

Ex: ped-al (pertaining to the feet or a foot); pedi-cure (care of the feet); pedo-graph (an imprint of the sole of the foot); pedo-motor (moving the foot).

foot (foot-like structure).

(Gr. *pous,* foot; genit. *podos*) -pod-; podi-; podo-; -podium; -podous.

Ex: pod-algia (pain in a foot); atelo-pod-ia (imperfect development of a foot); pod-alic (performed by the use of the feet); podo-gram (a print or outline of the foot); pseudo-podium (a foot-like part); plani-podous (having a flat foot).

force. See under *power.*

forehead (frontal).

(Gr. *metopon,* forehead) metopo-; metop-.

Ex: metop-odynia (pain in the region of the forehead); metopo-plasty (a plastic operation on the forehead or frontal bone). See also *front.*

foreign (foreign body; stranger).

(Gr. *xenos,* strange, foreign) xeno-.

Ex: xeno-genous (caused by the presence of a foreign body); xeno-menia (menstrual discharge from an abnormal place); xeno-phobia (an abnormal dislike for strangers).

foreign body. See under *foreign.*

form (shape; configuration).

(Gr. *eidos,* form) eid-; eido-.

Ex: eid-optometry (measurement of vision with regard to the perception of form); eido-logy (the study of form).

form (shape; configuration).

(Gr. *morphe,* form) morph-; -morph; morpho-; -morphy.

Ex: morph-allaxis (restoration of form); delo-morph-ous (having a definite form); morpho-logy (the study of forms); pseudo-morphy (condition of having an irregular form).

form (shape; image).

(L. *forma,* form) -form.

Ex: digiti-form (shaped like a finger); vermi-form (shaped like a worm); lingui-form (shaped like a tongue).

formation. See under *plastic surgery, process,* and *production.*

forth. See under *out.*

four.

(Gr. *tettares,* four) tetr-; tetra-.

Ex: tetra-brachius (a fetal monster having four arms); tetra-dactyly (the condition of having four digits); tetra-logy (a combination of four symptoms, conditions, etc.); tetr-atomic (composed of four atoms).

four (fourfold).

(L. *quadriplus,* fourfold) quadr-; quadri-.

Ex: quadr-angular (having four angles); quadri-ceps (having four heads); quadri-geminal (fourfold); quadri-para (a woman who had four childbirths); quadri-plegia (paralysis of all four limbs).

fraction. See under *part.*

fracture. See under *break.*

fragile (brittle).

(L. *fragilis,* fragile) fragil-; fragili-; fragilo-.

Ex: fragil-osis (condition marked by abnormal fragility); fragili-clinia (proneness to fragility); fragilo-cyte (fragile red blood cell).

fragrance. See under *odor.*

freezing. See under *cold.*

frenzy. See under *mania.*

friction. See under *rubbing.*

from (away from; off).

(L. *ab,* from) ab-.

Ex: ab-alienation (separation from sanity; mental derangement); ab-articular (away from a joint); ab-duct (to draw or move away from the median line); ab-enteric (away from the intestine); ab-errant (deviating from the normal place or course); ab-normal (away from normal; not normal); ab-rasion (a wearing away of tissue).

from (away from; down; off; reverse).

(L.) de-.

Ex: de-activate (make inactive); de-capitation; de-cerebrate (deprive of the cerebrum); de-compress (remove the pressure from); de-generate.

from (separation from; derivation from).

(Gr. *apo*, from) apo-.

Ex: apo-morphine (derived from morphine); apo-neurosis (from a sinew); apo-physis (an outgrowth from). See also *out*.

front (anterior; forehead).

(L. *frons*, forehead; genit. *frontis*) front-; fronti-; fronto-.

Ex: front-al (pertaining to the forehead; anterior); fronti-petal (moving to the front); fronto-parietal (pertaining to the frontal and parietal bones).

frontal. See under *forehead*.

frost. See under *cold*.

fructose. See under *fruit*.

fruit (fructose).

(L. *fructus*, enjoyment, fruit; *frux*, fruit) fruct-; fructi-; fructo-; frugi-.

Ex: fructi-vorous (eating mainly fruits); fruct-ose (fruit sugar); fructo-lysis (lysis of fructose); frugi-philous (fond of fruits).

function (performance).

(L. *fungi*, to perform; *functio*, performance) -funct-; function-.
Ex: function-al (involving the function of a part; capable of functioning); funct-ion; mal-function (impairment of function); hypo-function (decreased function).

fungus.

(L. *fungus*, fungus) fung-; fungi-; fungo-.

Ex: fung-ate (grow like a fungus); fungi-cide (a substance capable of destroying fungi); fungo-genic (encouraging the growth of fungi).

fungus (mushroom).

(Gr. *mykes,* fungus) myc-; mycet-; myceto-; myco-.

Ex: mycet-hemia (presence of fungi in the blood); myceto-genic (encouraging the growth of fungi); myco-dermatitis (dermatitis caused by infection with fungi); myc-osis (any disease caused by fungi).

funnel-shaped structure. See under *infundibulum.*

G

gallbladder.

(Gr. *chole,* bile, *kystis,* bladder) cholecyst-; cholecysto-.

Ex: cholecyst-ectomy (excision of the gallbladder); cholecyst-itis (inflammation of the gallbladder); cholecysto-pathy (disease of the gallbladder).

gallstone (biliary calculus).

(Gr. *chole,* bile; *lithos,* stone) cholelith-; cholelitho-.

Ex: cholelith-iasis (presence of gallstones in biliary tract); cholelitho-tomy (removal of gallstones through an incision).

galvanic electricity (direct current).

(Luigi *Galvani,* Italian physicist) galvan-; galvani-; galvano-.

Ex: galvan-ic (pertaining to electricity produced by a battery); galvani-zation (application of galvanic electricity, as in treatment); galvano-cautery (cautery utilizing direct current).

gamete (reproductive cell; malarial parasite).

(Gr. *gamete,* wife) gamet-; gameto-.

Ex: gamet-ic (pertaining to a gamete); gameto-genesis (the development of a male or female reproductive cell); gameto-cyte (a cell capable of producing gametes).

ganglion (group of nerve cells).

(Gr. *ganglion,* knot) gangli-; ganglio; ganglion-; gangliono-.

Ex: gangli-form (having the shape or form of a ganglion); ganglio-cyte (a cell of a ganglion); ganglion-ated (having a ganglion); gangliono-plegic (blocking the transmission through a ganglion).

gas. See under *air.*

gas in intestine (distention with gas).

(L. *flatus,* a blowing) flatul-; flatulo-.
Ex: flatul-ent (marked by the distention of the intestine with gas); flatulo-genic (causing flatulence); flatulo-lytic (relieving flatulence).

gel. See under *gelatin.*

gelatin (gel; jelly).

(L. *gelare,* to congeal) gelatin-; gelatino-; gelatini-.
Ex: gelatin-ase (an enzyme which decomposes gelatin); gelatini-ferous bearing gelatin; gelatino-lytic (dissolving gelatin). gelatino-lytic (dissolving gelatin).

genital organs of female.

(L. *pudere,* to be ashamed) pudend-; pudendi-; pudendo-.
Ex: pudend-algia (pain in the vulva); pudendo-plasty (a plastic operation on the female genital organs); pudendo-graphy (a description or pictorial representation of the female genital organs); pudendo-philia (keen interest in the female sex organs).

genus. see under *race.*

gigantic (huge; billion).

(Gr. *gigas,* giant; *gigantos,* huge) giga-; gigant-; giganto-.
Ex: giga-meter (one billion meters); gigant-ism (excessive size); giganto-cyte (a very large red blood cell).

give birth. See under *bear child.*

gland.

(Gr. *aden,* gland; genit. *adenos*) -aden-; adeni-; adeno-.
Ex: aden-algia (pain in a gland); aden-ectomy (excision of a gland); hyp-aden-ia (deficient activity of a gland); peri-aden-itis (inflammation of the tissue surrounding a gland); adeni-form (having the form of a gland); adeno-fibroma (a tumor composed of fibrous tissue and glandular structures).

gland.

(L. *glans,* an acorn; genit. *glandis*) gland-; glandi-; glandul-.
Ex: glandi-lemma (membrane surrounding a gland); glandul-ar (pertaining to a gland).

glass (glassy; translucent).

(Gr. *hyalos,* glass) hyal-; hyalo-.

Ex: hyal-in (a translucent albuminoid material); hyalo-phobia (fear of large plates of glass); hyal-oid (resembling glass).

globe. See under *ball.*

globulin. See under *ball.*

glomerulus of kidney.

(L. *glomus,* ball; *glomerulus,* diminutive of *glomus*) glom-; glomerul-; glomerulo-.

Ex: glomerul-itis (inflammation of glomeruli); glomerulo-nephritis (nephritis associated with inflammation of glomeruli).

glossy. See under *smooth.*

glucose (sweetness; sugar).

(Gr. *glykys,* sweet) gluc-; gluco-.

Ex: gluco-genesis (the formation of glucose); gluco-protein (a compound of a carbohydrate and a protein).

glue-like tissue.

(Gr. *glia,* glue) gli-; glia; glio-.

Ex: gli-oma (tumor composed of neuroglia); gli-osis (abnormal growth of neuroglia); gli-al (pertaining to neuroglia); neuro-glia (supporting structure or tissues of the nervous system); micro-glia (small cells of the neuroglia).

glycerin (glycerol).

(Gr. *glykeros,* sweet) glycer-; glycerin-; glycero-.

Ex: glycer-ide (an ester of glycerin); glycerin-ated (containing glycerin); glycero-philic (combining readily with glycerin).

glycerol. See under *glycerin.*

glycogen. See under *sugar.*

gnash (grind; gnaw; bite).

(Gr. brykein, gnash) brux-; bruxo-; brycho-.

Ex: brux-ism (grinding or gnashing of the teeth); bruxo-mania (neurotic gnashing of teeth); brychomania.

god (deity).

(Gr. *theos,* god) theo-.

Ex: theo-mania (a mental disorder in which the patient believes he is inspired by God); theo-phobia (fear of God); theo-morphism (the condition of having the image of God).

gonad (testicle; ovary).

(Gr. *gone,* seed) gonad-; gonado-.

Ex: gonad-ectomy (excision of a gonad); gonado-therapy (treatment with hormones from the ovary or testis); gonado-tropin (a substance which stimulates a gonad).

good (well; normal; easily).

(Gr. *eu,* well) eu-.

Ex: eu-angiotic (having a good supply of blood vessels); eu-genics (the study of the factors which may improve the race); eu-osmia (normal condition of the sense of smell).

grain, small. See under *granule.*

granule (grain; small particle).

(L. *granulum,* small grain) granul-; granuli-; granulo-.

Ex: granul-ation (the division of a substance into granules); granuli-form (having the shape of granules); granulo-cyte (a cell containing granules); granulo-plastic (producing granules).

gray matter of nervous system.

(Gr. *polios,* gray) polio-.

Ex: polio-clastic (destructive to the gray matter); polio-encephalopathy (any disease of the gray matter of the brain); polio-myelitis; polio-thrix (grayness of the hair).

great. See under *large.*

green (greenish; greenish yellow).

(Gr. *chloros,* green) chlor-; chlori-; chloro-.

Ex: chlor-emia ("green blood," i.e., chlorosis); chloro-phyll ("green leaf," i.e., the green pigment of leaves); chlor-opsia (green vision).

grind. See under *chew* and *gnash.*

grinding. See under *rubbing.*

groin (inguinal region).

(L. *inguen,* groin; genit. *inguinis*) inguin-; inguino-.

Ex: inguin-al (pertaining to the groin); inguino-scrotal (pertaining to the groin and the scrotum).

group of nerve cells. See under *nucleus of cell.*

growth. See under *development, increase,* and *tumor.*

gum.

   (L. *gingiva,* the gum) gingiv-; gingivo-.

   Ex: gingiv-ectomy (excision of a part of a gum); gingivo-labial (pertaining to the gums and the lips).

gyrus. See under *circle.*

H

habit. See under *condition.*

hair.

   (L. *pilus,* hair) -pil-; pilo-.

   Ex: de-pil-atory (a substance which removes hair); pilo-cystic (pertaining to a cyst containing hair); pilo-motor (capable of moving the hair); pilo-logy (the study of the hair with regard to growth, disorders, etc.).

hair (hairy). (Gr. *thrix,* hair; genit. *trichos*) tricho-.

   Ex: tricho-clasis (brittleness of the hair); tricho-genous (stimulating the growth of hair); tricho-logy (the study of hair); tricho-mycosis (infection of the hair with fungi).

half (less than usual).

   (L. *dimidius,* half) demi-.

   Ex: demi-facet (half of a facet); demi-lune (half moon); demi-monstrosity (partial malformation).

half (one half).

   (Gr.) hemi-.

   Ex: hemi-plegia (paralysis of half or one side of the body); hemi-sphere; hemi-anopia (defective vision in one half of the visual field); hemi-facial (affecting one side of the face).

half (partly; not fully).

   (L. *semis,* half) semi-.

   Ex: semi-canalis (a canal which is open on one side); semi-cartilaginous (partly of cartilage); semi-cretinism (partial cretinism); semi-lunar (resembling a half-moon).

hand (hand-like structure).

   (Gr. *cheir,* hand) cheir-; cheiro-; chir-; chiro-.

   Ex: cheir-algia (pain in the hand); cheiro-megaly (enlargement of a hand); cheiro-spasm (spasm of the muscles of a hand).

hand   (hand-like structure).

(L. *manus,* hand) -man-; mani-; manu-.

Ex: longi-man-ous (having long hands); mani-form (shaped like a hand); mani-pulate (to perform with the hand or hands); manu-script (a composition written by hand); manu-stupration (masturbation performed by hand).

hard   (fibrous; sclerous).

(Gr. *skleros,* hard) scler-; sclero-.

Ex: scler-adenitis (a hardening of a gland associated with inflammation); sclero-adipose (composed of both fibrous and fatty tissues); sclero-genic (causing a hardening of a tissue); scler-osis (an abnormal hardening).

hard (firm).

(L. *durus,* hard) -dur-; dura; dur-.

Ex: in-dur-ate (become hard); dura mater; dur-ematoma (hematoma of the dura mater); dura-plasty (plastic operation on the dura mater).

hard   (rocky; stony).

(L. *petra,* a rock) petri-; petro-.

Ex: petri-faction (the change to a stony or hard substance); petro-logy (the science of rocks); petro-philous (living on rocks).

hard palate. See under *palate.*

harlot. See under *prostitute.*

hate   (dislike; aversion).

(Gr. *misein,* to hate) mis-; miso-.

Ex: mis-andria (aversion for men); miso-gamy (a dislike for marriage); miso-neism (a dislike for change or new ways and ideas).

head   (uppermost part).

(Gr. *kephale,* head) cephal-; cephalo-.

Ex: cephal-algia (pain in the head); cephalo-metry (measurement of the head); cephalo-tomy (surgical cutting of the fetal head).

health. See under *hygiene.*

hearing.

(Gr. *akouein,* to hear) -acou-; -acous-; acoustico-; acousto-.
Ex: acou-esthesia (acoustic sensation); acou-meter (an instrument used to test the acuity of hearing); an-acous-ia (absence of hearing); acoustico-phobia (abnormal fear of sounds); acousto-gram (a tracing of sounds); ambly-acous-ia (dullness of hearing).

hearing (hear).

(L. *audire,* hear) audi-; audio-.
Ex: aud-ile (pertaining to hearing); audio-logy (the science of hearing); audio-visual.

heart (cardiac sphincter of stomach).

(Gr. *kardia,* heart) cardi-; cardio-.
Ex: cardi-algia (pain in the heart); cardi-ectasis (dilatation of the heart: cardio-centesis (surgical incision into the heart); cardio-hepatic (pertaining to the heart and the liver); cardio-neurosis (nervous disorder of the heart); cardio-spasm (spasm of the cardiac sphincter of the stomach).

heat.

(Gr. *therme,* heat) therm-; thermo-; -thermy.
Ex: therm-algesia (the production of pain by the application of moderate heat); thermo-biosis (the ability to thrive in a high temperature); thermo cautery (the use of heat in cautery), dia-thermy; hypo-thermy (low body temperature).

heat (warmth; fever).

(L. *calor,* heat) calor-; calori-.
Ex: calor-ic (pertaining to heat); calori-facient (producing heat); calori-meter (instrument for measuring amount of heat produced); calori-metry. See also *fever.*

heel.

(Gr. *pterna,* heel) ptern-; pterno-.
Ex: ptern-algia (pain in the heel); pterno-helcosis (ulceration of the heel); pterno-tomy (a surgical incision into the heel).

heel bone (calcaneus).

(L. *calx,* heel bone; *calcis*) calcane-; calcaneo-.
Ex: calcane-al (pertaining to the heel bone); calcaneo-cuboid

(pertaining to the calcaneus or heel bone and the cuboid);
calcaneus.

height (elevation).

(Gr. *hypsos,* height) hyps-; hypso-.

Ex: hypso-phobia (fear of being in or on a high place);
hypso-therapy (the utilization of high altitudes in the treatment of disease); hypso-kinetic (attaining considerable height).

hemoglobin.

(Gr. *haima,* blood; L. *globin,* a protein) hemoglobin-; hemo-
globini-; hemoglobino-.

Ex: hemoglobin-emia (presence of hemoglobin in the blood
plasma); hemoglobini-ferous (bearing hemoglobin); hemo-
globino-meter (an instrument used for determining the amount
of hemoglobin in the blood).

hemorrhoid.

(Gr. *haimorrhois,* hemorrhoid; pl. *haimorrhoides*) hemor-
rhoid-; hemorrhoidi-; hemorrhoido-.

Ex: hemorrhoid-ectomy (excision of hemorrhoids); hemor-
rhoid-al; hemorrhoid-algia (condition of having painful hemorrhoids); hemorrhoidi-form (shaped like a hemorrhoid); hem-
orrhoido-genic (conducive to the development of hemorrhoids).

hereditary.

(L. *heres,* heir; genit. *heredis*) heredo-.

Ex: heredo-diathesis (hereditary predisposition); heredo-im-
munity (hereditary immunity); heredo-pathia (an inherited
disease).

heredity.

(L. *hereditas,* heirship) heredit-.

Ex: heredit-able (capable of being inherited); heredit-ary;
heredit-y.

hermaphroditism.

(Gr. *Hermes,* Greek god; *Aphrodite,* Greek goddess of love)
hermaphrodit-.

Ex: hermaphrodit-ic (of the nature of a hermaphrodite, an
animal, plant or human possessing both male and female
reproduction organs); hermaphrodit-ism; hermaphroditi-smus.

high (aloft).

(Gr. *hypsi,* aloft) hypsi-; hyps-.

Ex: hypsi-cephaly (the condition of having a high skull); hypsi-gastria (condition of having the stomach placed high in the abdomen); hypsi-lophic (having a high crest or peak).

hernia (rupture; herniation).

(L. *hernia,* hernia) herni-; hernio-.

Ex: herni-ated (protruding in the form of a hernia); herni-clitic (inclined to be affected with a hernia); hernio-rrhaphy (an operation for the repair of a hernia).

hernia (tumor; swelling).

(Gr. *kele,* hernia) -cele.

Ex: adipo-cele (hernia containing fat); entero-cele (hernia containing a piece of intestine); recto-cele (hernia of the rectum).

herpes.

(Gr. *herpein,* to creep) herpes-; herpet-; herpeti-; herpeto-.

Ex: herpes-virus (the virus causing herpes simplex); herpet-ic; herpeti-form (resembling herpes); herpeto-genic (causing herpes).

hidden (concealed; secret).

(Gr. *kryptos,* hidden) crypt-; crypto-.

Ex: crypt-esthesia (subconscious perception); crypto-menorrhea (menstruation without an external discharge); crypto-toxic (having concealed toxic properties).

higher. See under *above.*

hip (hip joint).

(L. *coxa,* hip) cox-; coxi-; coxo-.

Ex: cox-algia (pain in the hip); cox-arthropathy (disease of the hip joint); coxo-femoral (pertaining to the hip and the thigh).

hip. See under *ischium.*

hollow (concave).

(Gr. *koilos,* hollow) koil-; koilo-.

Ex: koil-onychia (condition of having concave nails); koilo-sternia (condition of having a funnel chest).

hollow. See under *cavity.*

homosexual, female. See under *lesbian.*

honey (bee; sweet).

(Gr. *meli,* honey; *melissa,* bee) meli-; melisso-; melit-.

Ex: meli-biose (a kind of sugar); melisso-phobia (fear of bees); melit-ose (a sugar occurring in beets and other plant products).

horizontal posture. See under *bed.*

horny tissue (horn).

(Gr. *keras,* horn; genit. *keratos*) kerat-; keratin-; kerato-. *Ex*: kerat-ic (pertaining to horny tissue); keratin-ase (an enzyme which aids in the decomposition of keratin); keratoderma (thickening of the horny layer of the skin); keratolysis (peeling of the horny layer of the skin).

huge. See under *gigantic.*

humerus.

(L. *humerus,* shoulder) humer-; humero-.

Ex: humer-al (pertaining to the humerus); humero-radial (pertaining to the humerus and the radius); scapulo-humer-al (pertaining to the scapula and the humerus).

humidity. See under *moisture.*

humpback (kyphosis).

(Gr. *kyphos,* a hump) kyph-; kypho-; kyphot-.

Ex: kyph-osis (condition marked by a humped back); kyphoscoliosis (a condition marked by kyphosis and scoliosis); kyphot-ic (marked by kyphosis).

hundred (hundredth; hundredfold).

(L. *centum,* hundred) cent-; centi-.

Ex: cent-esimal (pertaining to divisions into hundredths); centi-grade (divided into 100 gradations); centi-normal (designating one hundredth of a normal or standard strength).

hundred (one hundred).

(Gr. *hekaton,* one hundred) hecto-.

Ex: hecto-liter (one hundred liters); hecto-cotylus (sexual arm of a cephalopod).

hunger (starvation).

(Gr. *limos,* hunger) lim-; limo-.

Ex: lim-asthenia (lack of strength due to hunger); limo-genous (caused by hunger); limo-therapy (treatment of disease by controlled hunger).

husk. See under *scale.*

hydatid (hydatid cyst).

(Gr. *hydatis,* watery vesicle; genit. *hydatidos*) hydatid-; hydatidi-; hydatido-.

Ex: hydatid-ectomy (excision of a hydatid cyst); hydatidiform (having the form of a hydatid cyst); hydatido-cele (a tumor containing hydatids).

hydrophobia. See under *rabies.*

hygiene (health).

(Gr. *hygieine,* of health) hygie-; hygio-; hygien-.

Ex: hygio-logy (science of hygiene or health); hygio-genesis (the establishment of conditions favorable to health); hygien-ist (a practitioner of hygiene).

hymen (membrane).

(Gr. *hymen,* membrane) hymen-; hymeno-.

Ex: hymen-ectomy (surgical excision of a hymen); hymenology (the study of membranes); hymen-atrophy (a wasting away or diminution of the hymen through a defect or failure in nutrition); hymeno-pachynsis (a thickening of the hymen).

hyoid bone (U-shaped).

(Gr. *hyoeides,* shaped like the letter upsilon) hyo-; hyoid-.

Ex: hyo-glossal (pertaining to the hyoid bone and the tongue); hyo-thyroid (pertaining to the hyoid bone and the thyroid gland); hyoid-ectomy (excision of the hyoid bone).

hypnotism. See under *sleep.*

hypophysis. See under *pituitary gland.*

I

icterus. See under *jaundice.*

idea (concept; impression).

(Gr. *idea,* appearance) ide-; idea-; ideo-.

Ex: ide-ation (formation of ideas); ideo-genetic (stimulating the formation of ideas); ideo-glandular (pertaining to the activity of glands which is initiated by a mental thought);

ideo-vascular (pertaining to vascular changes which result from certain thoughts or concepts).

identical. See under *equal.*

idleness.
(Gr. *thassein,* to sit idle) thass-; thasso-.
Ex: thasso-genous (caused by inactivity or idleness); thasso-phobia (fear of being idle or unoccupied); thasso-therapy (treatment of certain ailments by restricting the patient to idleness).

ileum (third part of small intestine).
(L. *ileum,* ileum) ile-; ileo-.
Ex: ile-ectomy (excision of the ileum); ile-itis (inflammation of the ileum); ileo-cecal (pertaining to the ileum and cecum); ileo-tomy (incision into the ileum).

ilium (flank).
(L. *ilium,* ilium) ili-; ilio-.
Ex: ili-ac (pertaining to the ilium); ilio-lumbar (pertaining to the flank and loin); ilio-costal (pertaining to the ilium and the ribs).

ill. See under *bad.*

illness. See under *disease.*

illumination. See under *light.*

illusory. See under *false.*

illustration. See under *image.*

image (picture; illustration).
(Gr. *eikon,* image) -eikon-; icon-; icono-.
Ex: anis-eikon-ia (inequality of the images in the two eyes); icono-lagny (sexual interest in pictures of nudes); icono-philia (uncommon fondness for pictures).

imitation (repetition; mimicry).
(Gr. *echo,* returned sound) echo-.
Ex: echo-lalia (repetition by patient of words addressed to him); echo-motism (repetition of the movements of others); echo-praxis (repetition by patient of physician's motions or of movements started by the physician with the patient's limbs).

immobility (adhesion; consolidation; ankylosis).

(Gr. *ankylosis,* stiffening) ankylo-; ankyl-.

Ex: ankylo-blepharon (adhesion of the eyelids); ankylo-dactylia (adhesion of digits); ankylo-glossia (a condition of tongue-tie); ankyl-osis (immobility of a joint); ankylo-poietic (causing immobility or consolidation of a joint).

immunity (resistance against; security from).

(L. *immunis,* exempt) immun-; immuni-; immuno-.

Ex: immuni-facient (producing immunity); immun-ization; immuno-therapy (medical treatment utilizing the phenomenon of immunity).

impaired. See under *difficult.*

imperforation. See under *adhesion.*

impression. See under *idea.*

improper (faulty; inadequate; bad; ill; wrong).

(L. *malus,* bad) mal-; male-.

Ex: mal-absorption (improper or inadequate absorption); mal-function (improper function); mal-formation (faulty formation); mal-nutrition (improper or inadequate nutrition).

in (into; on).

(L.) en-; em- (before *b, p,* and *m*).

Ex: en-capsulated (enclosed in a capsule); en-cephalon (the brain tissues situated in the cranium); en-gram (a lasting mark); em-pyema (accumulation of pus in a cavity of the body, especially the chest).

in (into; within; toward; on).

(L.) in-; il- (before letter *l*); ir- (before letter *r*); im- (before letters *m, p,* or *b*).

Ex: il-lusion; im-plantation (the insertion of something into); ir-rigation (washing with a stream of fluid); in-sufflation (the blowing of a medicinal substance into).

in back. See under *posterior.*

in direction of. See under *toward.*

in front. See under *before.*

inactive. See under *sleep.*

inadequate. See under *improper.*

incision (cut; depression; notch).

(L. *incidere,* to cut; pp. *incisus,* cut) incis-; inciso-.

Ex: incis-al (used in cutting); incis-ion; inciso-lingual (pertaining to the incisal and lingual aspects of a tooth).

incision. See under *cutting.*

inciting. See under *inducing.*

increase (growth; stimulation).

(Gr. *auxein,* increase) aux-; auxo-.

Ex: auxi-lytic (increasing the lytic effect); auxo-neurotropic (increasing the neurotropic properties).

increased. See under *more.*

incus (anvil-shaped).

(L. *incus,* anvil; genit *incudis*) incud-; incudo-; incudi-.

Ex: incud-al (pertaining to the incus); incudi-form (shaped like an incus or anvil); incudo-stapedial (pertaining to the incus and the stapes).

inducing (inciting; leading; stimulating).

(Gr. *agogos,* leading) -agogue.

Ex: emmen-agogue (an agent which induces or initiates menstruation); galact-agogue (a substance which promotes the production of milk in the breast); ptyal-agogue (a substance which stimulates the formation of saliva).

inducing (making; causing).

(L. *facere,* to make; *facientis*) -facient.

Ex: somni-facient (inducing sleep); parturi-facient (inducing labor); ithyphallo-facient (inducing erection of penis).

infant (young child).

(L. *infans,* infant; genit. *infantis*) infan-; infant-; infanti-; infanto-.

Ex: infan-cy; infanti-cide (the killing of an infant); infant-ile; infant-orium (a hospital for infants).

inflammation.

(Gr. *-itis,* inflammation; pl. *itides*) -itis; -itides.

Ex: bronch-itis (inflammation of bronchial tubes); neur-itis (inflammation of a nerve); appendic-itis; nephr-itides (all forms of nephritis).

inflammation.

(Gr. *phlox*, fire; genit. *phlogos*) phlog-; phlogo-.

Ex: phlog-istic (marked by inflammation); phlogo-cyte (a cell present in inflamed tissue); phlogo-genic (causing inflammation); phlogo-lytic (tending to resolve inflammation).

infundibulum (funnel-shaped structure).

(L. *infundibulum*, funnel) infundibul-; infundibuli-; infundibulo-.

Ex: infundibul-ar (pertaining to an infundibulum); infundibuli-form (shaped like an infundibulum or funnel); infundibulo-pelvic (pertaining to an infundibulum and pelvis of a kidney).

ingestion. See under *eating*.

inguinal region. see under *groin*.

injury (pain; hurt).

(L. *nocere*, to hurt) noci-.

Ex: noci-ceptive (capable of receiving stimuli caused by injury; receiving painful stimuli); noci-genic (causing injury); noci-fensive (serving to defend against injury).

injury. See under *trauma*.

inner. See under *inward* and *within*.

insanity (mental derangement).

(L. *luna*, moon) lun-; lunat-; lunato-.

Ex: lun-acy (insanity); lunat-ic; lunat-ism (the condition of being a lunatic); lunato-phobia (fear of insanity).

insect.

(L. *insectum*, insect)insect-; insecti-; insecto-.

Ex: insecti-cide (a substance which destroys insects); insecto-logy (the study of insects).

insects.

(Gr. *entomon*, insect) entom-; entomo-.

Ex: entomo-logy (the study of insects); entomo-philous (fond of insects; fertilized by pollen which is carried by insects).

inside. (within).

(L. *intra*, within) intra-.

Ex: intra-abdominal (within the abdomen); intra-cellular (within a cell or cells); intra-nasal (occurring inside the nose); intra-cranial (occurring within the cranium); intra-venous (within a vein).

inside See under *within.*

insufficient. See under *few.*

insulin.
(L. *insula,* island) insulin-; insulino-.
Ex: insulin-ase (an enzyme which inactivates insulin); insulino-genic (producing insulin).

intermediate. See under *middle.*

intervertebral disk. See under *disk.*

intestinal worm. See under *worm.*

intestine (small intestine).
(Gr. *enteron,* intestine) enter-; enteri-; entero-.
Ex: enter-ectomy (excision of a part of the intestine); enteri-form (shaped like an intestine); entero-centesis (surgical puncture of the intestine); entero-toxin (a toxin arising in the intestine).

intestine. See under *colon.*

into (inward; within; on the inside).
(L. *intro,* inwardly) intro-.
Ex: intro-mission (the introduction or insertion of one structure into another); intro-version (a turning of one's interests inward).

into. See under *in.*

inward (within; inner).
(Gr. *eso,* inward) eso-.
Ex: eso-ethmoiditis (inflammation within the ethmoid sinuses); eso-toxin (a toxin produced within the body); eso-tropia (a deviation of the eye inward, toward the midline).

inward. See under *into.*

iodine (iodide).
(Gr. *iodes,* violet-like) iod-; iodi-; iodino-; iodo-.
Ex: iod-emia (presence of iodides in the blood); iodi-metry (determination of the amount of iodine); iodino-phil (having an affinity for iodine); iodo-genic (producing iodine).

ion (cation; anion).

(Gr. *ienai,* to go) ion-; iono-; ionto-.

Ex: ion-ization; iono-genic (producing ions); ionto-phoresis (the introduction of ions into the tissues).

iris of eye (rainbow).

(Gr. *iris,* rainbow, iris; genit. *iridos*) ir-; irit-; irid-; iridi-; irido-.

Ex: ir-itis (inflammation of the iris); irid-ectomy (excision of part of the iris); iridi-form (shaped like the iris of the eye); irido-plegia (paralysis of the muscles of the iris).

iron.

(Gr. *sideros,* iron) sider-; sidero-.

Ex: Sidero-bacter (a genus of microorganisms having iron in the membranes); sidero-derma (a disorder caused by an abnormal metabolism of iron from hemoglobin); sidero-penia (a deficiency of iron).

iron (steel; ferrous; ferric).

(L. *ferrum,* iron) ferr-; ferri- (for iron in trivalent form); ferro- (for iron in divalent form).

Ex: ferr-ated (impregnated within iron); ferri-cyanide (a compound of iron and cyanide); ferro-protein(a compound of iron and protein).

irregular (varied in shape).

(Gr. *poikilos,* varied) poikilo-.

Ex: poikilo-cyte (a red blood cell having an irregular shape); poikilo-derma (a mottled appearance of the skin); poikilo-thermic (having a body temperature which varies with the environment).

ischium (hip).

(Gr. *ischion,* hip) ischi-; ischio-.

Ex: ischi-algia (pain in the hip); ischio-femoral (pertaining to the ischium and the femur); ischio-pubic (pertaining to the ischium and the pubic bone).

isthmus (connecting structure).

(Gr. *isthmos,* narrow passage) isthm-; isthmo-.

Ex: isthm-ectomy (excision of an isthmus, especially of the thyroid gland); isthm-itis (inflammation of an isthmus); isthmo-spasm (spasm of an isthmus, as of the fauces).

itching.

(L. *prurire,* to itch) prurit-; prurito-.

Ex: prurit-ic (pertaining to, or marked by, itching); prurito-genous (caused by itching); prurito-genic (causing itching or pruritus).

J

jaundice (icterus).

(Gr. *ikteros,* jaundice) icter-; ictero-.

Ex: icter-ic (pertaining to jaundice); icter-itious (affected by jaundice); ictero-hepatitis (inflammation of the liver associated with jaundice).

jaw (jawbone).

(Gr. *gnathos,* jaw) gnath-; gnatho-.

Ex: gnath-odynia (pain in the jaw); gnatho-plasty (a plastic operation on the jaw); a-gnath-ia (absence of the lower jaw); pro-gnath-ism (projecting jaw).

jejunum.

(L. *jejunum,* empty) jejun-; jejuno-.

Ex: jejun-ectomy (excision of a part of the jejunum); jejun-itis (inflammation of the jejunum); jejuno-stomy (the formation of an opening in the wall of the jejunum).

join (unite).

(L. *jungere,* to join; pp. *junctus*) junct-.

Ex: con-junct-iva (membrane covering the eyeball); con-junct-ure (a joining together); junct-ion; dis-junct-ion (act of separating).

joined (junction).

(Gr. *zygon,* yoke) zygo-; zyg-.

Ex: zyg-apophysis (an articular process of a vertebra); zygo-dactyly (a fusion of digits); zygo-spore (a spore formed by the union of two gametes).

joint (articulation).

(Gr. *arthron*) arthr-; arthri-; arthro-.

Ex: arthr-itis (inflammation of a joint); arthro-centesis (puncture of a joint); arthro-pathy (joint disease); arthro-plasty. See also *articulation.*

juice. See under *chyle.*

junction. See under *joined.*

K

keen. See under *sharp.*

ketone (ketone bodies).

(Gr. *keton,* acetone) keto-; keton-.

Ex: keto-genic (producing ketones); keto-lysis (the splitting of ketones); keton-ization (conversion into ketones).

kidney (ren).

(Gr. *nephros,* kidney; *nephritikos,* nephritic) nephr-; nephrit-; nephro-.

Ex: nephr-itis (inflammation of a kidney); nephr-ectomy (surgical removal of a kidney); nephrit-ic (pertaining to the kidneys; pertaining to nephritis); nephrito-genic (causing nephritis).

kidney (ren).

(L. *ren,* kidney; pl. *renes*; genit. *renis*) ren-; reni-; reno-.
Ex: ren-al (pertaining to the kidneys); reni-cardiac (pertaining to the kidneys and the heart); reni-puncture (a surgical puncture of the capsule of the kidney); reno-pathy (any disease of the kidneys); reno-tropic (having a special effect on the kidneys).

kill (killer; killing).

(L. *caedere,* kill) -cide; -cid-.

Ex: bacteri-cid-al (capable of killing bacteria); spermato-cide (substance capable of killing spermatozoa); sui-cide (act of killing oneself).

knee.

(Gr. *gone,* knee) gon-; gone-; gony-.

Ex: gon-arthritis (inflammation of the knee or knee joint);
gone-itis (inflammation of a knee); gony-campsis (an abnormal bending of the knee).

knee (knee joint).

(L. *genu,* knee) genu-.

Ex: genu-al (pertaining to the knee); genu-cubital (pertaining to the knees and elbows); genu-pectoral (resting on, or
pertaining to, the knees and the chest).

kneecap. See under *patella.*

knowledge (recognition; appreciation).

(Gr. *gnosis,* knowledge) -gnosia; -gnosis; -gnostic.

Ex: a-gnosia (inability to recognize sensory stimuli); diagnosis; baro-gnosis (the ability to recognize weight); pro-
gnostic (a symptom or sign helpful in making a prognosis).

kyphosis. See under *humpback.*

L

labium. See under *lip.*

labium minus (lust).

(L. *nympha,* labium minus) nymph-; nympho-.

Ex: nymph-ectomy (excision of the labia minora); nymph-itis
(inflammation of the labia minora); nympho-hymeneal (pertaining to the labia minora and the hymen); nympho-mania
(keen sexual desire in a female).

labor. See under *childbirth.*

laborious. See under *difficult.*

lacrimal apparatus. See under *tears.*

lacrimal gland.

(Gr. *dakryon,* a tear; *aden,* gland) dacryaden-; dacryoaden-;
dacryoadeno-.

Ex: dacryoaden-algia (pain in a lacrimal gland); dacryoden-
oma (a tumor of the lacrimal gland).

lacrimal sac.

(Gr. *dakryon,* a tear; *kystis,* sac) dacryocyst-; dacryocysti-; dacryocysto-.

Ex: dacryocyst-ectasia (dilatation of a lacrimal sac); dacryocysti-tome (instrument for cutting into the lacrimal sac); dacryocysto-cele (herniation of a lacrimal sac).

lactic. See under *milk.*

lamella (thin plate; scale; layer).

(L. *lamella,* small lamina) lamell-; lamelli-.

Ex: lamell-ar (pertaining to lamellae); lamell-ate (consisting of lamellae); lamelli-branch (a kind of mollusk); lamelli-form (having the form of a lamella); lamelli-rostal (pertaining to birds having lamellae in the bill).

lamina (thin plate; layer).

(L. *lamina,* thin plate) lamin-; lamino-; lamina-.

Ex: lamin-ated (composed of laminae); lamin-ectomy (excision of a lamina of a vertebra); lamina-graphy (body section roentgenography).

large (big; one million).

(Gr. *megas,* big) meg-; mega-.

Ex: mega-colon (a large colon); mega-karyocyte (a large cell occurring in bone marrow); mega-cycle (an electrical unit of one million cycles per second); meg-ohm (a unit of one million ohms).

large (great; big; powerful).

(Gr. *megas,* large) megal-; megalo-.

Ex: megal-encephalon (an abnormally large encephalon); megalo-blast (a large erythroblast); megalo-clitoris (an abnormally large clitoris).

large (long; enlarged).

(Gr. *makros,* long, large) macr-; macro-.

Ex: macr-adenous (having a large gland or glands); macro-cephalous (having a large head); macro-phage (a large phagocytic cell); macro-scopic (large enough to be seen without a microscope).

larynx   (laryngeal).
   (Gr. *larynx,* larynx; genit. *laryngos*) laryng-; laryngo-.
   Ex: laryng-itis (inflammation of the larynx); laryngo-pathy (a disease of the larynx); laryngo-scopy (inspection of the larynx).

lasting. See under *long.*

later. See under *after.*

law (usage; custom).
   (Gr. *nomos,* law) nom-; nomo-.
   Ex: nomo-tropic (following the law or normal course); nomo-genesis (evolution in accordance with a predetermined law); nomo-topic (occurring in the usual place).

layer. See under *lamella* and *lamina.*

lead (conduct; convey).
   (L. *ducere,* to lead) duct-; ducti-; duc-; -duct.
   Ex: ab-duct (lead away); con-duct; ab-duc-ent (abducting; moving away); duct-us; duct-ule; duct-ile (capable of being drawn out).

leading. See under *inducing.*

leaf (leaf-like structure).
   (Gr. *phyllon,* leaf) -phyll-; phyllo-.
   Ex: chloro-phyll (the green pigment of plants); phyllo-porphyrin; phyllo-genetic (producing leaves); phyllo-morphous (having the shape of a leaf); phyllo-taxy (the distribution of leaves).

left (left side).
   (L. *sinister,* left) sinistr-; sinistro-.
   Ex: sinistr-ad (toward the left); sinistr-aural (designating a person who hears better with the left ear); sinistro-cerebral (pertaining to the left side of the cerebrum).

left (to the left; on the left).
   (L. *laevus,* left) levo-; levul-.
   Ex: levo-rotation (rotation to the left); levo-duction (a turning of the eye to the left); levul-ose (a levorotatory sugar).

leg (leg-like structure; shin).
   (L. *crus,* leg; genit. *cruris*) crur-; cruri-; cruro-.
   Ex: crur-al (pertaining to the leg); brachio-crur-al (pertaining

to the arm and leg); cruro-femoral (pertaining to the leg and thigh).

lens (crystalline lens of eye).

(L. *lens*, lentil; genit. *lentis*) lens-; lent-; lenti-; lento-; lenticul-.

Ex: lens-o-meter (an instrument to measure lenses); lent-itis (inflammation of the crystalline lens); lenti-conus (abnormal protrusion on surface of crystalline lens); lenticul-ar (pertaining to a lens).

lens (crystalline lens of eye).

(Gr. *phakos*, a lentil) phac-; phaco-.

Ex: phaco-cele (a herniation of the crystalline lens); phaco-planesis (abnormal mobility of the crystalline lens); phaco-meter (an instrument used to measure the refractive power of lenses).

leprosy.

(Gr. *lepra*, leprosy) lepr-; lepra-; lepro-.

Ex: lepra-phobia (fear of leprosy); lepr-oma (a lesion of leprosy); lepro-logy (study of leprosy).

lesbian (female homosexual).

(Gr. *Lesbos*, island in Aegean) lesb-; lesbi-; lesbio-; lesbo-.

Ex: lesb-ian (pertaining to female homosexuality); lesb-iatria (medicine dealing with female homosexuality); lesbi-clinia (a tendency toward female homosexuality); lesbio-phobia (fear of, or aversion for, female homosexuals); lesbo-gnomonic (indicative of female homosexuality).

less (little; decrease).

(Gr. *meion*, less) mio-; mi-; miot-.

Ex: mio-lecithal (containing little yolk); mi-osis (decrease in size of the pupil); miot-ic (causing contraction of the pupil); colpo-mi-osis (decrease in the size of the vagina).

less than normal. See under *beneath*.

lethargy. See under *stupor*.

leukocyte (white blood cell).

(Gr. *leukos*, white; *kytos*, cell) leukocyt-; leukocyto-; leucocyt-.

Ex: leukocyt-uria (the presence of leukocytes in the urine); leukocyt-hemia (a form of leukemia); leukocyto-lysis (a lysis of white blood cells); leukocyto-penia (a decrease in the number of leukocytes in the blood).

level. See under *even.*

libido. See under *sexual desire.*

lie in bed. See under *bed.*

life.

(L. *vita,* life) -vit-; vita-; vital-.

Ex: re-vital-ize (to restore to life or to a viable condition); de-vital-ize (to deprive of life; to deprive of the nerve supply); vit-amin; vita-scope (an instrument for the study of animal movements).

life (living; involving living matter).

(Gr. *bios,* life) bio-.

Ex: bio-assay (assay involving the use of experimental animals); bio-chemistry (chemistry of living organisms or matter); bio-logy (the science of living organisms); bio-psy (removal and examination of a specimen from the living body).

ligament (band; bundle).

(Gr. *desmos,* band) desm-; desmio-; desmo-.

Ex: desm-ectasis (abnormal stretching of a ligament); desm-itis (inflammation of a ligament); desm-oid (resembling a ligament; fibroid); desmo-logy (study of ligaments).

ligament (ligamentum).

(L. *ligamentum,* binder) ligament-; ligamento-.

Ex: ligament-ectomy (excision of a ligament); ligamento-pexy (fixation of a ligament); ligament-ous (of the nature of a ligament).

light (illumination).

(L. *lumen,* light; genit. *luminis*) lumi-; lumin-; lumini-; lumino-.
Ex: lumi-flavin (a luminiferous decomposition derivative of riboflavin); il-lumin-ation; lumin-escence (the process of giving off light without appreciable heat); lumini-ferous (conveying light); lumino-phore (a chemical group which imparts the property of luminescence to the molecule).

light (illumination).

(L. *lux,* light; *lucere,* to shine) luci-.

Ex: luci-fugal (shunning light); luci-petal (seeking light); luci-ferase (an enzyme which initiates bioluminescent activity).

light (photograph).

(Gr. *phos,* light; genit. *photos*) phos-; photo-.

Ex: phos-genic (producing light); photo-electric (pertaining to electricity produced or controlled by light); photo-phobia (intolerance of light); photo-tropism (movement of an organism in response to light).

lightning.

(Gr. *keraunos,* lightning) kerauno-.

Ex: kerauno-neurosis (a neurosis initiated or aggravated by fear of lightning or by a stroke of lightning); kerauno-phobia (abnormal fear of lightning).

like. See under *resembling.*

liking. See under *loving.*

limb (extremity).

(Gr. *melos,* limb) -mel-.

Ex: mel-algia (pain in the limbs or a limb); caco-mel-ia (congenital deformity of a limb); aniso-mel-ia (inequality in the size of the limbs).

limb (extremity; end; tip).

(Gr. *akron,* extremity) acro-.

Ex: acro-dermatitis (dermatitis affecting the hand or feet); acro-genous (growing at the tip); acro-geria (a premature aging of the skin of the extremities); acro-megaly (hyperplasia of the extremities); acro-mycosis (mycosis affecting the extremities).

lime. See under *calcium.*

lip (edge; margin; brim).

(Gr. *cheilos,* lip) cheil-; cheilo-.

Ex: cheil-itis (inflammmation of a lip); cheil-ectomy (excision of a lip or part thereof); cheilo-plasty (plastic surgery on a lip); cheilo-rrhaphy (suturing of a lip).

lip (lip-like structure).

(L. *labium,* lip) lab-; labi-; labio-.

Ex: labi-al (pertaining to a lip); labi-form (shaped like a lip); labio-dental (pertaining to the lips and the teeth); labiolingual (pertaining to a lip and the tongue); labio-plasty (a plastic operation on a lip).

liquid (fluid).

(L. *liquidus,* fluid; *liquere,* to be liquid) lique-; liqui-; liquid-. *Ex*: lique-facient (causing to liquefy); liqui-form (in the form of a liquid); Liquid-ambar (a genus of trees).

little. See under *few* and *less.*

liver.

(Gr. *hepar,* liver; genit. *hepatos*) hepat-; hepatico-; hepato-. *Ex*: hepat-ectomy (excision of a portion of the liver); hepatico-enterostomy (the formation of an anastomosis between a hepatic duct and the intestine); hepato-genic (forming liver tissue); hepato-lith (a calculus formed in the liver).

living. See under *alive.*

living matter. See under *life.*

lobe (projecting part; subdivision).

(L. *lobus,* lobe) lob-; lobo-. *Ex*: lob-ar (pertaining to, or involving, a lobe); lob-ate (composed of lobes); lob-ectomy (excision of a lobe); lobo-tomy (a surgical cut into a lobe).

lobule (lobulus).

(L. *lobulus,* small lobe) lobul-. *Ex*: lobul-ar (pertaining to, or involving, lobules); lobul-ose (composed of lobules); lobul-ated.

loin (lumbar).

(L. *lumbus,* loin) lumb-; lumbar-; lumbo-. *Ex*: lumb-ar (pertaining to the loins); lumbar-ization; lumbo-costal (pertaining to, or involving, the loin and the ribs); lumbo-sacral (pertaining to the lumbar region and the sacrum). See also *flank.*

long (elongated).

(Gr. *dolichos,* long) dolicho-. *Ex*: dolicho-cephalic (having a long head); dolicho-facial (having a long face); dolicho-morphic (having a long and slender build).

long (lasting; durable).

(L. *longus,* long) long-; longi-.

Ex: long-evity (condition of living long); longi-lineal (having a long, narrow build); longi-pedate (having long feet).

louse (lice).

(L. *pediculus,* louse) pedicul-; pediculi-; pediculo-.

Ex: pedicul-ar (pertaining to lice); pedicul-osis (condition of being infested with lice); pediculi-cide (a substance which destroys lice); pediculo-phobia (fear of lice).

love, sexual. See under *sexual desire.*

loving (liking; preferring; having an affinity for).

(Gr. *philein,* to love; *philos,* loving) -phil-; phila-; -phile; -philia; philo-; -philous; -philus- -phily.

Ex: andro-phil-ous (having a predilection for men); phila-letia (an abnormal desire for death); baso-phile (staining with a basic dye); hemo-philia; philo-neism (love for change or novelty); dendro-philous (preferring trees); Haemo-philus (microorganism growing best on blood); thermo-phily (a preference for high temperatures).

low temperature. See under *cold.*

lower jaw. See under *chin* and *mandible.*

lumbar. See under *loin.*

lung.

(L. *pulmo,* lung; genit. *pulmonis*) pulmo-; pulmon-; pulmono-.

Ex: pulmo-gram (an x-ray picture of the lungs); pulmo-metry (the measurement of the capacity of the lungs); pulmon-ecto-my (excision of a lung); pulmon-itis (inflammation of a lung); pulmono-hepatic (pertaining to the lungs and the liver); pulmono-logy (the study of the lungs).

lung (air; breath).

(Gr. *pneumon,* lung) pneumo-; pneumon-; pneumono-.

Ex: pneumo-angiography (roentgenography of the blood vessels of the lung); pneumo-coniosis (a disease of the lung caused by inhalation of dust); pneumon-ectomy (surgical removal of a lung); pneumon-itis (inflammation of a lung); pneumono-centesis (the surgical puncture of a lung); pneumo-thorax (an accumulation of gas in the space between the pleurae).

lust. See under *sexual desire.*

lutein. See under *corpus luteum.*

lymph (lymphatic system).

(L. *lympha,* fluid) lymph-; lymphat-; lymphati-; lymphato-; lympho-.

Ex: lymph-edema (swelling due to presence of an excessive amount of lymph); lymphato-logy (study of lymph); lympho-cyte; lymphati-ostomy (the making of an opening in a lymphatic duct).

lymph node.

(L. *lympha,* fluid; Gr. *aden,* gland) lymphaden-; lymphadeno-

Ex: lymphaden-ectomy (excision of a lymph node); lymphaden-itis (inflammation of a lymph node); lymphadeno-pathy (any disease of lymph nodes).

lymph vessel.

(L. *lympha,* fluid; Gr. *angeion,* vessel) lymphangi-; lymphangio-; lymphang-.

Ex: lymphangi-ectomy (excision of a lymph vessel); lymphang-itis (inflammation of a lymph vessel); lymphangi-oma (a tumor of lymph vessels); lymphangio-plasty (plastic surgery on lymph vessels).

lymphatic system. See under *lymph.*

M

maimed (deformed).

(Gr. *peros,* maimed) pero-.

Ex: pero-brachius (a fetus having deformed arms); pero-cephalus (a fetus having a deformed head); pero-mania (a mania to deform or maim).

making. See under *inducing* and *production.*

making, process of

(L. *facere,* to make) -faction.

Ex: albe-faction (the process of making white); putre-faction (decomposition of organic matter by bacteria, etc.); cale-faction (the act of making warm or hot); rube-faction (process of making red).

male (masculine).

(L. *vir,* man; *virilis,* manly) -vir-; viril-; virili-; viri-.
Ex: vir-ile (strongly masculine); viril-escence (development of male characteristics); viril-ia (male reproductive organs); viril-ism (masculinity in a female); viril-ization (development of male characteristics in a female); viri-potent (sexually potent).

male. See under *man* and *masculine.*

male ancestor. See under *father.*

male generative power. See under *penis.*

malignancy. See under *cancer.*

malleolus (*pl.* malleoli).

(L. *malleus,* hammer; *malleolus,* little hammer) malleol-; malleoli-; malleolo-.
Ex: malleol-ar (pertaining to, or involving, malleoli or a malleolus); malleoli-form (having the shape of a malleolus); malleolo-tomy (a surgical cutting into a malleolus).

malleus (largest auditory ossicle).

(L. *malleus,* a hammer) malleo-.
Ex: malleo-incudal (pertaining to the malleus and the incus); malleo-tomy (a surgical cutting of the malleus, as in ankylosis of the ossicles).

mammary gland. See under *breast.*

man (male; masculinity).

(Gr. *aner,* man; genit. *andros*) andr-; andri-; andro-.
Ex: andr-ase (a hypothetical male hormone); andri-form (resembling a male or a male structure); andro-gen (a masculinizing substance); andro-gynism (female pseudohermaphroditism); andro-morphous (marked by a masculine appearance); andro-sterone (an androgenic substance).

man. See under *male.*

mandible (lower jawbone).

(L. *mandibulum,* a jaw) mandibul-; mandibuli; mandibulo-.
Ex: mandibul-ar (pertaining to the mandible); mandibuli-form (shaped like the mandible); mandibulo-temporal (pertaining to the mandible and the temporal bone).

mania (craving; frenzy).

(Gr. *mania,* madness) -mania-.

Ex: mania-phobia (fear of being affected by a mania); photo-mania (a craving for sunlight); pyro-mania (mania for arson); gyneco-mania (excessive craving for women).

manifest. See under *visible.*

manly. See under *masculine.*

many (much; several; excessive).

(Gr. *polys,* many) poly-.

Ex: poly-adenitis (inflammation of several glands); poly-arthritis (inflammation of several joints); poly-phagia (excessive eating); poly-phobia (the condition of having many fears).

many (multiple; much).

(L. *multus,* many) multi-.

Ex: multi-cellular (consisting of many cells); multi-fidus (divided into several parts); multi-glandular (involving many glands).

many. See under *several.*

margin. See under *lip.*

marriage (sexual union).

(Gr. *gamos,* marriage) gam-; gamo-; -gamy.

Ex: gamo-genesis (production of offspring in marriage; sexual reproduction); gamo-phobia (fear of marriage); endo-gamy (marriage within one's tribe or group); poly-gamy.

marrow (bone marrow).

(L. *medulla,* marrow) medull-; medullo-.

Ex: medull-ary (pertaining to bone marrow); medull-itis (inflammation of marrow); medull-ization (formation of marrow); medullo-culture (a bacterial culture containing marrow).

marrow (bone marrow).

(Gr. *myelos,* marrow) myel-; myelo-.

Ex: myel-itis (inflammation of bone marrow); myelo-cyte (a cell of the marrow); myelo-genous (originating in bone marrow).

marrow. See also *medulla.*

masculine (male; manly).

(L. *masculus,* male) -mascul-; masculin-; masculo-.

Ex: e-mascul-ate (to deprive of masculine characteristics); masculin-ization (acquisition of male characteristics); masculo-nucleus (the male pronucleus).

masculine. See under *male.*

masculinity. See under *man.*

mass. See under *tumor.*

massage (knead; rub).

(Fr. *masser,* to massage; Gr. *massein,* to knead) mass-; masso-.

Ex: masso-therapy (treatment by means of massage); masso-genic (inducing massage or massage-like stimulation); mass-ataraxia (relaxation produced by massage).

masticate. See under *chew.*

mastoid cells. See under *mastoid process.*

mastoid process (mastoid antrum; mastoid cells).

(Gr. *mastoeides,* resembling a breast or nipple) mastoid-; mastoideo-; mastoido-.

Ex: mastoid-algia (pain in the mastoid process); mastoid-ectomy (excision of the mastoid process or the mastoid cells); mastoideo-centesis (surgical puncture of the mastoid cells); mastoido-tomy (a surgical incision into the mastoid process).

material. See under *matter.*

matter (substance; material).

(Gr. *hyle,* matter) hyl-; hyle-; hylo-.

Ex: hylo-genesis (the genesis or formation of matter); bio-hylo-tropic (affecting living matter); bio-hylo-genous (derived from living matter); hetero-hyl-ous (of a different substance).

maxilla (bone of upper jaw).

(L. *maxilla,* jawbone) maxill-; maxillo-.

Ex: maxill-ary (pertaining to the maxilla); maxill-ectomy (excision of a part of the maxilla); maxillo-mandibular (pertaining to the maxilla and the mandible).

mean. See under *middle.*

measure (measurement).

(Gr. *metron,* measure) metr-; metro-; -metry.

Ex: metro-logy (the science of weights and measures); psycho-metry (measurement of psychic processes with regard to duration); calori-metry (measurement of heat absorbed or given off); pelvi-metry (measurement of the pelvic dimensions).

meatus (opening; passage).

(L. *meatus,* passage) meat-; meato-.

Ex: meat-al (pertaining to a meatus); meato-meter (an instrument for measuring a meatus); meato-tomy (a surgical cutting of a meatus).

medial. See under *middle.*

median. See under *middle.*

medicinal substance. See under *drug.*

medicine. See under *drug* and *physician.*

medulla (inner part of organ).

(L. *medulla,* marrow) medull-; medulla-; medullo-.

Ex: medull-ary (pertaining to a medulla); medull-ectomy (excision of the medulla of an organ); medulla-centesis (surgical puncture of a medulla); medullo-adrenal (pertaining to the medulla of the adrenal glands).

medulla spinalis. See under *spinal cord.*

melanin. See under *black.*

membrana tympani. See under *eardrum.*

membrane (thin layer of tissue).

(L. *membrana,* membrane) membran-; membrani-; membrano-.

Ex: membran-aceous (having the structure or nature of a membrane); membrani-form (having the form of a membrane); membrano-cartilaginous (pertaining to membrane and cartilage). See also *hymen.*

memory (remembrance).

(Gr. *mnasthai,* to remember; *mnemon,* remembering) mnem-; mnemon-; -mnesia; -mnesis.

Ex: a-mnesia (absence of memory); mnemon-ics (the study of memory); hypo-mnesis (weak memory); hyper-mnesis (a better than normal memory).

meninges (membranes).

 (Gr. *meninx,* membrane; genit. *meningos*) mening-; meninge-; meningeo-; meningi-; meningo-.

 Ex: mening-itis (inflammation of the meninges); meninge-al (pertaining to the meninges); meningeo-rrhaphy (surgical suture of the meninges); meningi-oma (a tumor of the meninges); meningo-pathy (any disease or disorder of the meninges).

menses. See under *menstruation.*

menstruation (menses; month).

 (Gr. *men,* month; genit. *menos;* L. *mensis,* month) men-; meno-; menstru-.

 Ex: men-arche (the beginning of the menstrual function); meno-pause (the end of the menstrual function); menstru-ation; meno-phobia (fear of menstruation); meno-rrhagia (excessive menstrual flow); dys-meno-rrhea (painful menstruation).

mental condition. See under *mind.*

mental derangement. See under *insanity.*

mercury (mercurous; mercuric).

 (L. *mercurius,* mercury; *hydrargyrum,* mercury) mercur-; mercuri-; mercuro-; hydrargyr-; hydrargyro-.

 Ex: mercur-ammonium (pertaining to, or involving, ammonia and mercury); mercuri-al (pertaining to mercury); mercur-ic (pertaining to mercury having a valence of two); mercur-ous (pertaining to mercury having a valence of one); hydrar-gyro-mania (a mental disorder caused by mercury poisoning).

microscopic. See under *small.*

middle (medial; mean).

 (L. *medius,* middle) medi-; medio-; mid-.

 Ex: medi-frontal (pertaining to the middle of the frontal bone); medi-sect (to divide or cut in the middle); medio-lateral (pertaining to the middle and the side); mid-section (a cut or cutting through the middle).

middle (intermediate; median).

 (Gr. *mesos,* middle) mes-; mesi-; mesio-; meso-.

 Ex: mes-encephalon (the midbrain); mesi-al (pertaining to the middle); mesio-buccal (pertaining to the mesial surface and buccal surface of a tooth); meso-derm (the middle layer of the embryo).

middle ear. See under *tympanum.*

middle position. See under *neutral.*

milk

(Gr. *gala,* milk; genit. *galaktos*) galact-; galacta-; galacto-.

Ex: galact-acrasia (abnormal condition of milk formation in the breast); galacto-phagous (subsisting on milk); galacto-poietic (producing milk).

milk (lactic).

(L. *lac,* milk; genit. *lactis*) lact-; lacti-; lacto-.

Ex: lact-acidase (an enzyme producing lactic acid fermentation); lact-agogue (a substance stimulating the secretion of milk); lacti-vorous (subsisting mainly on milk); lacto-genic (stimulating the secretion of milk in the breast).

million. See under *large.*

millionth. See under *small.*

mind (emotions; soul).

(Gr. *thymos,* mind) -thymia; thymo-.

Ex: thymo-genic (caused by emotion); thymo-pathy (any mental disorder); cyclo-thymia (manic depressive condition); lypo-thymia (mental depression).

mind (mental).

(L. *mens,* mind; genit. *mentis*) -ment-; menti-.

Ex: de-ment-ia (a form of mental deterioration); a-ment-ia (subnormal mental development); ment-al; menti-metry (measurement of mental capacity).

mind (mental condition).

(Gr. *phren,* mind) -phren-; phreno-.

Ex: hebe-phren-ia (a type of mental disorder); schizo-phren-ia; phreno-logy; phreno-pathy (any disorder of the mind).

mind (mental condition; psyche).

(Gr. *psyche,* soul, mind) psych-; psycho-.

Ex: psych-asthenia (a type of neurosis marked by anxiety, etc.); psycho-analysis (analysis of the mind); pyscho-delic; psycho-pathic (affected by mental illness); psych-osis (a serious mental illness); psycho-therapy (treatment of mental disorders by suggestion, reassurance, etc.).

missiles (projectiles).

(Gr. *ballein,* to throw) ballist-; ballisto-.
Ex: ballist-ics (scientific study of the motion of missiles); ballisto-phobia (abnormal fear of missiles).

moisture (dampness; humidity; fluid).

(Gr. *hygros,* wet) hygr-; hygro-.
Ex: hygr-ectasia (expansion caused by moisture); hygr-oma (a mass or tumor formed by an accumulation of fluid); hygro-meter (an instrument for determining the amount of moisture in the air); hygro-phobia (fear of, or sensitivity to, dampness).

monster, fetal.

(Gr. *teras,* monster; genit. *teratos*) terat-; terato-.
Ex: terat-ism (the condition of being a fetal monster); terato-genesis (the development of a fetal monster); terat-oid (resembling a monster); terato-logy (the study of monsters and fetal malformation).

month. See under *menstruation.*

more (increased; excess).

(Gr. *pleion,* more) pleio-; pleo-.
Ex: pleio-chromia (increased pigmentation); pleio-tropy (the quality of manifesting itself in a variety of ways); pleo-cytosis (an increase in the number of cells); pleo-nectic (combining with more than the average amount of oxygen). See also *several.*

more than normal. See under *excessive.*

mother (motherhood).

(L. *mater,* mother; *maternus,* maternal) matern-; materno-; matro-; matri-.
Ex: matern-al (pertaining to, or derived from the mother); matern-ity (the condition of being a mother); materno-hemo-therapy (treatment with mother's blood); matro-clinous (having characteristics derived from the mother); matri-cide (the murder of a mother by her child).

motion (movement).

(Gr. *kinema,* motion; genit. *kinematos*) kine-; kinemat-; kinemato-; cinemat-; cinemato-.

Ex: kine-scope (an instrument for measuring the refraction of the eye); kinemat-ics (the study of motion); kinemato-graph (an instrument showing pictures of objects in motion); cinemat-ization (amputation forming a stump suitable for motion).

motion (movement).

(L. *kinesis,* motion) cine-; -cine.

Ex: cine-micrography (the making of motion pictures through a microscope); auto-cine-sis (movement originating within the organism).

motion. See under *bearing* and *movement.*

motor. See under *movement.*

mouth (opening).

(L. *os,* mouth; genit. *oris*) or-; -or; oro-.

Ex: or-ad (directed toward the mouth); or-al (pertaining to the mouth); peri-or-al (surrounding the mouth); per-or-al (by way of the mouth); oro-lingual (pertaining to the mouth and the tongue); oro-pharynx; oro-nasal (involving the mouth and the nose).

mouth (opening; pore).

(Gr. *stoma,* mouth; genit. *stomatos*) -stom-, stomat-; stomato-; -stomy.

Ex: ozo-stom-ia (bad odor from the mouth); atelo-stom-ia (imperfect development of the mouth); stomat-algia (pain in the mouth); stomato-rrhagia (bleeding from the mouth).

movement (motion; motor).

(L. *movere,* to move; pp. *motus*) mot-; moto-; motor-; motoro-.
Ex: mot-ile (capable of moving); moto-facient (causing motion); motor-icity (the capability to move or cause motion); motoro-germinative (producing, or developing into, muscles).

movement (motion; movable).

(Gr. *kinein,* move; *kinesis,* movement; *kinetos,* movable) kin-; kine-; kinemat-; kines-; kinesio-; kineto-; kino-.

Ex: kine-plasty (plastic surgery aiming to maintain movement) kinemat-ics (the study of the mechanics of motion); kines-algia (pain induced by movement); kinesio-logy (the study of motion of living organisms); kineto-genic (producing movement); kino-meter (an instrument to measure displacement, as of the uterus).

moving toward (seeking).
(L. *petere,* to seek) -petal.
Ex: centri-petal (seeking or moving toward the center); cortici-petal (moving toward the cortex); acro-petal (seeking the top); nucleo-petal (moving toward a nucleus).

much. See under *many.*

mucin. See under *mucus.*

mucous tissue. See under *mucus.*

mucus (mucin).
(L. *mucus,* fluid covering mucous membranes) muc-; muci-; mucin-; mucino-; muco-.
Ex: muc-ase (an enzyme which aids in the decomposition of mucin); muci-ferous (bearing or producing mucus); mucin-emia (presence of mucin in the blood); mucino-gen (a substance regarded as a precursor of mucin); muco-purulent (composed of mucus and pus).

mucus (mucous tissue).
(Gr. *myxa,* mucus) myx-; myxo-.
Ex: myx-adenitis (inflammation of a mucous gland); myxo-chondroma (a tumor composed of mucous tissue and cartilaginous tissue); myx-oma (a tumor composed of mucous tissue); myxo-poiesis (the formation of mucus).

multiple. See under *many.*

murder. See under *kill.*

muscles (muscle tissue).
(Gr. *mys,* a muscle; genit. *myos*) my-; myo-.
Ex: my-algia (pain in a muscle); my-asthenia (muscular weakness); leio-my-oma (a tumor of smooth muscle); myo-cardium (the muscular layer forming the wall of the heart); myo-fibroma (tumor composed of muscle tissue and fibrous tissue).

mutation (transformation; change).

(L. *mutare,* to change) mut-; muta-.

Ex: mut-ase (an enzyme which stimulates certain chemical reactions); muta-gen (an agent producing change or mutation); muta-rotation (a certain transformation of isomers).

mutual. See under *between.*

myelin (myelin sheath).

(Gr. *myelos,* marrow) myelin-; myelino-.

Ex: myelin-ization (the process of being covered with myelin); myelino-geny (the formation of myelin); myelin-osis (any disease or disorder of myelin).

N

nail (fingernail; toenail; claw).

(Gr. *onyx,* nail; genit. *onychos*) onych-; onycho-.

Ex: onych-ectomy (excision of a nail); onycho-malacia (abnormal softening of the nails); onycho-mycosis (fungus infection of the nails).

naked (uncovered; exposed).

(Gr. *gymnos,* naked) gymno-.

Ex: gymno-scopophilic (fond of viewing the naked body); gymno-sophy (nudism); gymno-phobia (an aversion for the naked body).

name (term; word; nomenclature).

(Gr. *onoma,* name; genit. *onomatos*) onomato-.

Ex: onomato-logy (the science of names or terminology); onomato-mania (a mental disorder involving names or words); onomato-phobia (fear of certain names or words).

name (title; nomenclature).

(Gr. *onyma,* name) -onym; -onymic; -onymous; -onymy.

Ex: ep-onym (name of a substance, condition, etc., based on the name of a person); top-onym (name of a region); organ-onymy (the naming of organs); taut-onymic (in a binomial system, having both names the same).

naris. See under *nostril.*

narrow (contracted; little).

(Gr. *stenos,* narrow) steno-.

Ex: steno-cephaly (abnormal narrowness of the head); steno-peic (having a narrow slit); steno-stomia (narrowness of the mouth); steno-thermic (able to live only in a narrow range of temperature).

narrow. See under *slender.*

narrowing. See under *stricture.*

nativity. See under *birth.*

nature (natural; physical agents; facial expression).

(Gr. *physis,* nature) phys-; physic-; physico-; physio-.

Ex: phys-iatrics (treatment by the use of physical agents); physic-ian; physico-genic (caused by physical agents); physio-logic (natural); physio-gnomy (the judgment of mental characteristics by the facial expression); physio-lysis (a natural disintegration).

navel (omphalus).

(Gr. *omphalos,* navel) omphal-; omphali-; omphalo-.

Ex: omphal-ectomy (surgical excision of the navel); omphal-itis (inflammation of the navel); omphalo-rrhagia (bleeding from the navel); omphali-form (shaped like, or resembling, a navel).

navel. See under *umbilicus.*

near (close to; beside).

(L. *juxta,* near) juxta-.

Ex: juxta-articular (near a joint); juxta-glomerular (close to a glomerulus); juxta-spinal (near the spine). See also *to.*

nearest (closest).

(L. *proximus,* next) proxim-; proximo-.

Ex: proxim-al (closer or closest to a particular point of reference); proximo-buccal (pertaining to the proximal surface and buccal surface of a tooth).

neck (cervix).

(Gr. *trachelos,* neck) trachel-; trachelo-.

Ex: trachel-ectomy (excision of the cervix); trachel-odynia (pain in the neck); trachelo-logy (the study of the neck); trachelo-tomy (the cutting of the neck of the uterus).

neck   (cervix of uterus).

   (L. *cervix,* neck; genit. *cervicis*) cervic-; cervico-.
   Ex: cervic-al (pertaining to the neck or the cervix); cervic-
   ectomy (excision of the cervix of the uterus); cervico-facial
   (pertaining to the neck and the face); cervico-vaginitis (inflammation of the cervix and the vagina).

neck   (throat).

   (L. *jugulum,* neck) jugul-.
   Ex: jugul-ar (pertaining to the neck); jugul-ation (strangu-
   lation).

needle   (pointed object).

   (L. *acus,* needle) acu-.
   Ex: acu-closure (the closure of a cut or laceration by means
   of a surgical needle); acu-pressure (the checking of a hemorrhage from a cut artery by the use of needles in the adjacent
   tissues); acu-puncture (surgical puncture with a needle).

negative.   See under *not* and *without.*

neither.   See under *neutral.*

nematode   (thread).

   (Gr. *nema,* thread; genit. *nematos*) nemat-; nemato-; nematod-.
   Ex: nemat-helminth (a thread-like worm); nemato-cide (an
   agent which kills nematode worms); nematod-iasis (infestation
   with nematode worms).

neoplasm.   See under *tumor.*

nerve   (nervous system; nervous tissue; nervus).

   (Gr. *neuron,* nerve, sinew) neur-; neuro-.
   Ex: neur-asthenia (weakness or exhaustion of nerves); neur-
   ectomy (excision of a nerve); neuri-noma (a tumor arising
   from the sheath of a nerve); neuro-glia (supporting structure
   of the nervous system); neuro-toxin (a toxin which is especially
   destructive to nerve tissue).

nerve   (nervous system; nervus).

   (L. *nervus,* nerve, cord) nerv-; nervi-; nervo-.
   Ex: nerv-al (pertaining to a nerve); nervi-motion (motion produced by the stimulation of a nerve); nervo-muscular (pertaining to nerves and muscles).

nervous system. See under *nerve.*

net. See under *rete.*

network. See under *rete* and *reticulum.*

neutral (neither; middle position).

(L. *neutralis,* neutral) neutro-; neutr-.

Ex: neutro-cyte (a cell stainable by neutral dyes); neutr-on (a fundamental particle of an atom bearing no electrical charge); neutro-phil (designating a structure stainable by neutral dyes).

new (recent; strange; foreign).

(Gr. *neos,* new) ne-; neo-.

Ex: ne-arthrosis (new or false joint); neo-blastic (derived from new tissue); miso-ne-ism (aversion for new things).

new (fresh; recent).

(Gr. *kainos,* new) cen-; ceno-.

Ex: ceno-genesis (appearance of new features); ceno-phobia (fear of new things).

next to. See under *after.*

night (darkness).

(L. *nox,* night; genit. *noctis*) noct-; nocti-; nocto-.

Ex: noct-albuminuria (the presence of albumin in the urine produced during the night); noct-ambulation (sleep walking); nocti-phobia (fear of the night); nocto-phoria (the condition of being more alert and functional at night).

night (darkness).

(Gr. *nyx,* night; genit. *nyctos*) nyct-; nycti-; nycto-.

Ex: nyct-algia (pain occurring especially at night); nyct-alopia (the inability to see properly at night or in partial darknness); nycti-tropic (changing position at night, as certain plants); nycto-hemeral (pertaining to both night and day).

nipple.

(Gr. *thele,* nipple) thel-; thele-; thelo-.

Ex: thel-algia (pain in a nipple); thele-plasty (a plastic operation on a nipple); thel-itis (inflammation of a nipple).

nipple (nipple-like structure).

(L. *mamilla,* teat) mamill-; mamilla-; mamilli-.

Ex: mamill-ary (pertaining to a nipple or nipples); mamilli-

form (having the shape of a nipple); mamill-itis (inflammation of a nipple).

nipple-like projection. See under *papilla.*

nitrates. See under *nitrogen.*

nitrogen (nitrates; nitrites).

(Gr. *nitron,* niter) nitr-; nitri-; nitro-; nitrit-.

Ex: nitr-amine (a nitro compound of an amine); nitri-fication
(the process of combining with nitrogen); nitrit-oid (similar
to a nitrite); nitro-bacterium (a microorganism which converts
ammonia into nitrites); nitro-meter (an apparatus to measure
the amount of nitrogen produced during a chemical reaction).

no. See under *none* and *not.*

nomenclature. See under *name.*

none (nothing; no).

(L. nullus, none) nulli-; nollo-.

Ex: nulli-gravida (a woman who has never been pregnant);
nulli-para (a woman who has borne no children); nulli-gamist
(a person who has never been married).

normal (correct; straight).

(Gr. *orthos,* straight) orth-; ortho-.

Ex: orth-ergasia (normal function or work); ortho-chromatic
(having the normal color); ortho-pedics; orth-optics (a method
of eye exercises); ortho-static (induced by standing erect or by
standing).

normal (usual; conforming to rule).

(L. *norma,* rule) norm-; norma-; normo-.

Ex: norm-ergic (performing in the normal manner); normo-
calcemia (a normal level of calcium in the blood); normo-
cyte (a normal red blood cell); normo-trophic (having a normal development).

normal. See under *good.*

nose.

(Gr. *rhis,* nose; genit. *rhinos*) rhin-; rhino-.

Ex: rhin-edema (swelling of the nose); rhin-itis; rhino-genous
(originating in the nose); rhino-kyphosis (condition of having
a humped nose); rhino-scopy (examination of the nose).

nose (nasus).

(L. *nasus,* nose) nas-; naso-.

Ex: nas-itis (inflammation of the nose); naso-palatine (pertaining to the nose and the palate or palatine bone); naso-pharynx.

nostril (naris).

(L. *naris,* nostril) nar-; nari-; nario-.

Ex: nari- ectasis (abnormal dilatation of a nostril); intra-narial (situated within a nostril); nario-plasty (a plastic operation on a nostril).

not (negative).

(L. *non,* not) non-.

Ex: non-antigenic (having no antigenic properties); non-viable (not capable of surviving); non-nucleated (not having a nucleus).

not (negative; reversal).

(ME) un-.

Ex: un-balanced (not having the normal balance); un-conscious; un-official (not listed in the U.S.P., N.F., etc.); un-organized (having no definite or constant structure); un-saturated; un-striated (having no striae).

not (no; without).

(L.) in-; il- (before letter *l*); ir- (before letter *r*); im- (before letters *m, p,* or *b*).

Ex: in-animate (not alive); in-compatible (not in agreement); ir-reversible (that cannot be reversed); im-perforate (not perforated); il-legitimate. See also *without.*

not fully. See under *half.*

notch. See under *incision.*

nothing. See under *none.*

nourishment. See under *nutrition.*

nucleus (nut; kernel).

(Gr. *karyon,* nut) kary-; karyo-.

Ex: kary-apsis (the joining of nuclei); karyo-cyte (a cell having a nucleus); karyo-genesis (the formation of a nucleus); karyo-lytic (destructive to nuclei).

nucleus of cell (group of nerve cells; central element).

(L. *nucelus,* nucleus; *nux,* nut; genit. *nucis*) nucle-; nucleo-; nuclei-.

Ex: nucle-ic (pertaining to, or occurring in, nuclei); nuclei-form (shaped like a nucleus); nucle-osis (an increase in the formation of nuclei); nucleo-toxin (a toxin affecting nuclei).

nude (bare; uncovered).

(L. *nudus,* nude) nud-; nudi-; nudo-.

Ex: nudi-phobia (an aversion for nudity); nudo-mania (a strong desire to be naked); nud-oneiria (persistent dreams involving nudity); nudo-graphia (description of nudity).

nutrition (nourishment; food).

(L. *nutrire,* nourish) nutri-; nutrio-; nutrition-.

Ex: nutri-torium (the nitritional system of the body); nutrio-logy (the study of nutrition and food); nutrition-ist (a person learned in nutrition).

nutrition (nourishment; food).

(Gr. *trophe,* food) -troph-; tropho-; -trophy.

Ex: myo-troph-ic (nourishing to muscle tissue); tropho-cyte (a cell which supplies nourishment to another cell); tropho-neurosis (a nervous disease caused by defective nutrition); tropho-therapy (treatment by regulation of the food intake); osteo-trophy (the nourishment of bone).

nystagmus (nodding; oscillation).

(Gr. *nystagmos,* drowsiness; *nystazein,* to nod in sleep) nystagm-; nystagmi-; nystagmo-.

Ex: nystagm-ic (pertaining to nystagmus); nystagmi-form (resembling nystagmus); nystagmo-genic (producing nystagmus).

O

observing. See under *viewing.*

occiput of cranium.

(L. *occiput,* back of skull) occipit-; occipito-.

Ex: occipit-al (pertaining to the occiput); occipit-alization (an abnormal union between the occipital bone and the atlas);

occipito-frontal (pertaining to the occiput and the frontal bone or forehead).

occurring before. See under *before.*

odor (aroma; fragrance).
(L. *odor,* odor) odori-; odoro-.
Ex: odori-ferous (bearing an odor); odori-metry (the measurement of the intensity of odors); odoro-graphy (a learned description of odors).

odor. See under *smell.*

off. See under *from.*

oil (oleum).
(L. *oleum,* oil) ole-; oleo-.
Ex: ole-ase (an enzyme occurring in olive oil); oleo-therapy (treatment of disease with oil); oleo-thorax (the injection of oil into the chest, between the layers of the pleura). See also *fat.*

old (early; primitive; first).
(Gr. *palaios,* old) pale-; paleo-.
Ex: pale-encephalon (the old or ancient brain); paleo-cortex (the older portion of the cortex of the brain); pale-ontology (the study of early forms of life).

old age.
(Gr. *presbys,* old) presby-.
Ex: presby-cusis (the impairment of hearing characteristic of old age); presby-opia (the hyperopia and impairment of vision characteristic of old age).

old age (aged person; elderly man or woman).
(Gr. *geras,* old age; *geron,* old man; genit. *gerontos*) ger-; gerat-; geri-; gerio-; gero; geronto-.
Ex: gerat-ic (pertaining to old age); ger-iatric (pertaining to the treatment of the elderly); geri-odontics (dentistry dealing with the problems of the aged); gerio-psychosis (mental disorder characteristic of old age); gero-derma (dystrophy of the skin observed in the aged); gero-morphism (premature appearance of old age); geronto-philia (fondness for old persons).

olecranon of ulna.

(Gr. *olekranon,* olecranon) olecran-; olecrano-.

Ex: olecran-oid (resembling an olecranon); olecran-al (pertaining to the olecranon); olecrano-humeral (pertaining to the olecranon and the humerus).

oleum. See under *oil.*

omentum (omentum majus; omentum minus).

(L. *omentum,* omentum) oment-; omenti-; omento-.

Ex: oment-ectomy (excision of an omentum or a part thereof); oment-itis (inflammation of an omentum); omento-pexy (an operation in which the greater omentum is attached to another tissue or organ).

omphalus. See under *navel.*

on (upon; over; outside; beside).

(Gr. *epi,* on) ep-; epi-; eph- (before an h).

Ex: ep-arterial (above an artery); eph-emeral (over the day; lasting only a day); epi-condyle (bony eminence above a condyle); epi-nephros (adrenal gland); epi-phyte (a plant organism growing as a parasite on another plant).

one. (L. *unus,* one) uni-.

Ex: uni-articular (pertaining to one joint); uni-focal (having one focus); uni-lateral (pertaining to one side); uni-cellular (composed of one cell).

one (single; alone).

(Gr. *monos,* one) mon-; mono-.

Ex: mon-arthric (involving one joint); mon-esthetic (pertaining to one sense); mono-mania (mental derangement about one subject); mono-nuclear (having a single nucleus).

one and a half.

(L. *sesqui-,* more by a half) sesqui-.

Ex: sesqui-basic (designating a substitution of two atoms of a base for three hydrogen atoms of an acid); sesqui-alteral (one and a half times as large as another).

one fourth. See under *quarter.*

one-tenth (tenth; tenth part).

(L. *decem,* ten) deci-.

Ex: deci-gram (tenth part of a gram); deci-liter; deci-meter;

deci-normal (having one tenth of the concentration of a normal solution).

one thousandth (one thousand).

(L.*mille,* thousand) milli-.

Ex: milli-ampere (one thousandth part of an ampere); milli-meter (one thousandth part of a meter); milli-second (one thousandth of a second).

one's own. See under *personal* and *same.*

oneself. See under *self.*

opening. See under *meatus, mouth,* and *ostium.*

opposed to. See under *against.*

opposite (contrary to; against; complementary).

(L. *contra,* against) counter-.

Ex: counter-irritation (an irritation which opposes another irritation); counter-traction (traction which opposes another traction). See also *against.*

opsonin.

(Gr. *opsonein,* to buy provisions) opsino-; opson-; opsono-; opsoni-.

Ex: opsino-gen (a substance which stimulates the formation of opsonins); opsoni-fication (the process of making bacteria susceptible to the activity of phagocytes); opsono-metry (the determination of the amount of opsonin present).

optic. See under *vision.*

optic nerve. See under *optics.*

optics See under (optic nerve; eye; sight).

(Gr. *optikos,* pertaining to sight) optic-; optico-.

Ex: optic-al (pertaining to optics or sight); optico-ciliary (pertaining to the optic and ciliary nerves); optico-kinetic (pertaining to, or involving, movement of the eyes).

orbit (eye socket; orbita).

(L. *orbita,* path) orbit-; orbito-.

Ex: orbit-al (pertaining to the orbit); orbito-nasal (involving the orbit and the nose); orbito-tomy (a surgical cutting into the orbit).

order. See under *arrangement.*

organ (organum).

(Gr. *organon,* organ) organ-; organo-.

Ex: organ-icism (a theory of organic disease); organo-genesis (the development of organs); organ-oid (resembling an organ); organo-therapy (treatment by the use of animal organs or organ extracts). See also *viscera.*

orientation. See under *arrangement.*

orifice. See under *ostium.*

original. See under *earliest* and *primitive.*

originate. See under *produce.*

oscillate (fluctuate; swing).

(L. *oscillare,* to swing) oscill-; oscillo-.

Ex: oscillo-graph (an instrument used to record electrical variations or oscillations); oscillo-meter (an instrument used to measure oscillations).

osmosis (impulse).

(Gr. *osmos,* impulse) osmo-; osmoso-.

Ex: osmo-logy (the study of osmosis); osmo-philic (designating a solution which is subject to osmosis); osmoso-logy (the study of osmosis).

ossicle (small bone).

(L. *ossiculum,* a small bone) ossicul-; ossiculo-.

Ex: ossicul-ectomy (excision of an ossicle); ossiculo-tomy (the incision or cutting into an ossicle).

ostium (orifice; opening).

(L. *ostium,* an opening) osti-; -ostial; ostio-.

Ex: osti-ary (pertaining to an ostium); inter-ostial (situated between two openings); ostio-stenosis (the narrowing of an ostium).

other (another; abnormal; reversal).

(Gr. *allos,* other) all-; allo-.

Ex: all-ergy (abnormal work or reaction); allo-biosis (a condition of abnormal or reversed reactivity); allo-erotism (sexual desire directed toward another); allo-plasty (the use of grafts taken from sources other than the human body).

other (another; different).

> (Gr. *heteros,* other) heter-; hetero-.
>
> *Ex*: heter-csthcsia (condition of having different sensations in adjoining regions of the skin); hetero-cellular (composed of different types of cell); hetero-cyclic (containing atoms of different elements); hetero-nomous (pertaining to different laws of growth); hetero-sexual (pertaining to the other or opposite sex).

other side. See under *across.*

out (from; forth; away from; thoroughly; without).

> (Gr. *ex,* out) ex-; ef- (before *f*); e- (before *b, d, g, h, l, m, n, r, v*); ec- (before *c, s*); es- (before words of French origin).
>
> *Ex*: ex-acerbation (intensification of the severity of a disease); ex-anthem (an eruption or breaking out); ex-cavation (a hollowing out); ex-cision (act of cutting out); ex-crescence (an outgrowth); ex-crete (throw out); ex-hale (breathe out); ex-pectorate (spit out); ex-tract (to draw out); e-duct (draw or lead out); ec-dysis (a throwing off or shedding); es-cape (to get out or away).

out (without; from).

> (L.) e-; ec-.
>
> *Ex*: e-bonation (removal of bone fragments); ec-bolic (throwing out; oxytocic); ec-centric (out of the center); ec-chondroma (growth from surface of cartilage); ec-chymosis (a pouring out of blood); ec-thyma (pustular eruption or breaking out).

outer. See under *outside.*

outer layer. See under *cortex.*

outside (external).

> (L. *exter,* outside) exter-; extro-.
>
> *Ex*: extero-ceptive (receiving stimuli from the external environment); extero-fective (responding to stimuli from the external environment).

outside (external; outer).

> (Gr. *ektos,* outside) ecto-.
>
> *Ex*: ecto-derm (the external of the three layers of the embryo);

ecto-plasm (outer portion of the cytoplasm); ecto-zoon (parasite living on the external surface of the host).

outside (outward; external; outer).

(Gr. *exo,* outside) exo-.

Ex: exo-cardial (situated outside the heart); exo-crine (secreting outside or outwardly); exo-dontics (dentistry dealing
with the extraction of teeth); exo-toxin (a toxin found outside the microorganism producing it).

outside of (beyond; in addition).

(L. *exter,* outside) extra-; extro-.

Ex: extra-articular (outside a joint); extra-cellular (outside of
a cell); extra-dural (outside the dura mater); extra-vasation
(a flow, as of blood, from a vessel to the outside); extra-
uterine (situated outside the uterus); extro-vert (person whose
interests are turned outward).

outward. See under *outside.*

ovary (ovarium).

(Gr. *oophoron,* ovary; *oon,* egg; *pherein,* to bear) oophor-;
oophoro-.

Ex: oophor-algia (pain in an ovary); oophor-ectomy (excision
of an ovary); oophor-itis (inflammation of an ovary); oophoro-
tomy (a surgical cutting into the ovary); oophor-rhagia (bleeding from an ovary).

ovary (ovarium).

(L. *ovarium,* ovary) ovario-; -ovari-.

Ex: ovario-centesis (a surgical operation in which the ovary
is punctured); ovario-genous (arising in the ovary); ovario-
hysterectomy (the surgical removal of the ovaries and the
uterus); par-ovari-an (situated near an ovary).

over. See under *above, excessive,* and *on.*

ovule (young ovum).

(L. *ovulum,* ovule) ovul-; ovulo-.

Ex: ovul-ation (the discharge of an ovule from the ovary);
ovulo-genic (producing ovules); ovulo-genous (developing
from an ovule).

ovum (egg).

> (L. *ovum,* egg) ovi-; ovo-.
> *Ex*: ovi-duct (a duct serving as a passage for ova); ovi-form (shaped like an egg); ovi-parous (laying eggs from which the young organisms are hatched outside the body); ovo-genesis (the production of ova).

ovum. See under *egg.*

ovum, young. See under *ovule.*

oxidation. See under *oxygen.*

oxygen (oxidation).

> (Gr. *oxys,* acid) -ox-; oxi-; oxid-; oxy-; oxygen-.
> *Ex*: an-ox-emia (lack of oxygen in the blood); hyp-ox-ia (a deficiency of oxygen in a tissue); oxi-meter (instrument for measuring the oxygen saturation of the blood); oxid-ase (an enzyme which stimulates oxidation); oxy-hemoglobin (a compound of oxygen and hemoglobin); oxy-purine (a purine containing oxygen as a part of the molecule); oxygen-ation (the process of providing or saturating with oxygen).

oxyurid. See under *pinworm.*

P

pain (ache).

> (Gr. *algos,* pain) alge-; algesi-; -algia; algo-.
> *Ex*: alge-donic (involving both pleasure and pain); algesi-meter (an instrument used to measure sensitivity to pain); my-algia (pain in a muscle); hyper-algia (excessive sensitivity to pain); algo-genic (inducing pain).

pain (ache; discomfort).

> (Gr. *odyne,* pain) odyn-; odyno-; -odynia.
> *Ex*: odyn-acusis (a condition in which sound causes pain); odyno-meter (an instrument for measuring degrees of pain); odyno-phobia (an abnormal fear of pain). See also *injury.*

painful. See under *difficult.*

paint (picture; depict).

> (L. *pingere,* to paint; pp. *pictus*) pict-; picto-.
> *Ex*: picto-graph (a picture chart used to test vision); picto-

phrenia (excessive mental visualization); picto-therapy (the use of painting as a means of therapy or relaxation).

palate (hard pallate; soft palate).

(Gr. *ouranos,* roof of mouth) uranisco-; urano-.
Ex: uranisco-lalia (a speech defect caused by a cleft palate); urano-plasty (a plastic operation on the palate); urano-schism (the condition of having a cleft palate); urano-plegia (paralysis of the muscles of the soft palate).

palate (palatum; roof of mouth).

(L. *palatum,* palate) palat-; palati-; palato-.
Ex: palat-al (pertaining to the palate); palati-form (shaped like the palate); palato-glossal (pertaining to the palate and the tongue); palato-pharyngeal (pertaining to the palate and the pharynx).

palm of hand.

(L. *palma,* palm) palm-; palmi-; palmo-.
Ex: palm-ar (pertaining to the palm); palm-esthetic (felt in the palm); palmi-form (resembling the palm); palmo-scopy (diagnostic inspection of the palm).

palpate. See under *touch.*

palpebra. See under *eyelid.*

pancreas.

(Gr. *pan,* all; *kreas,* flesh) pancreat-; pancreatico-; pancreato-; pancreo-.
Ex: pancreat-ectomy (excision of the pancreas or a part thereof); pancreatico-splenic (pertaining to the pancreas and the spleen); pancreato-tropic (having a special influence on the pancreas); pancreo-zymin (an enzyme which stimulates the pancreas).

papilla (small nipple-like projection).

(L. *papilla,* small elevation) papill-; papilli-; papillo-.
Ex: papill-ectomy (surgical excision of a papilla); papill-itis (inflammation of a papilla); papilli-form (shaped like a papilla); papillo-retinitis (inflammation of the optic papilla and the retina).

papule (pimple).

(L. *papula,* pimple) papul-; papuli-; papulo-.

Ex: papul-ation (formation of papules); papuli-ferous (bearing papules); papulo-vesicular (pertaining to both papules and vesicles).

paralysis (stroke; blow).

(Gr. *plege,* a stroke) -plegia.

Ex: quadri-plegia (paralysis of all four limbs); cyclo-plegia (paralysis of the ciliary muscles); entero-plegia (paralysis of the intestine); para-plegia (paralysis of the lower half of the body); mono-plegia (paralysis of one limb).

parasitic worm. See under *worm.*

part (segment; fraction).

(Gr. *meros,* part) mer-; meri-; mero-.

Ex: mer-ergasia (part disorder; mild mental disorder); mer-ism (a pattern of structure in which similar parts are repeated); meri-spore (a spore produced by the segmentation of another spore); mero-diastolic (involving part of the diastole).

particle, small. See under *granule.*

partition. See under *septum.*

partly. See under *half.*

parturition. See under *childbirth.*

passage. See under *meatus.*

patella (kneecap).

(L. *patella,* small pan) patell-; patella-; patelli-; patello-.

Ex: patell-ectomy (excision of a patella); patella-pexy (surgical fixation of the patella); patelli-form (shaped like a patella); patello-tibial (pertaining to the patella and the tibia); infra-patell-ar (situated below the patella).

pathway (nerve path).

(Gr. *hodos,* path) hod-; hodo-.

Ex: hodo-tomy (the surgical cutting of a nerve pathway); hodo-logy (the study of the pathways of the nervous system).

pecular to. See under *personal.*

peduncle (stem; stalk).

(L. *pedunculus,* small foot, stalk) peduncul-; pedunculi-; pedunculo-.

Ex: peduncul-ated (provided with a peduncle); peduncul-ectomy (excision of a peduncle); pedunculi-form (shaped like a peduncle); pedunculo-tomy (a surgical cutting of a cerebral peduncle).

pellagra.

(L. *pellis,* skin; Gr. *agra,* seizure) pellagr-; pellagra-; pellagri-; pellagro-.

Ex: pellagr-oid (a disorder resembling pellagra); pellagra-phobia (fear of pellagra); pellagri-form (resembling pellagra); pellagro-logy (the study of pellagra).

pelvis.

(L. *pelvis,* a basin) pelv-; pelvi-; pelvio-; pelvo-.

Ex: pelv-ic (pertaining to the pelvis); pelvi-meter (an instrument used for measuring the pelvis); pelvio-peritonitis (inflammation of the peritoneum lining the pelvis); pelvo-spondylitis (inflammation of the pelvic portion of the vertebral column).

pelvis of kidney.

(Gr. *pyelos,* pelvis) pyel-; pyelo-.

Ex: pyel-ectasis (dilatation of the pelvis of the kidney); pyel-itis; pyelo-cystitis (inflammation of the pelvis of the kidney and of the bladder); pyelo-gram (an x-ray picture of the pelvis of the kidney and of the ureter); pyelo-nephritis (inflammation of the kidney and the kidney pelvis).

penis.

(L. *penis,* tail, phallus) pen-; peni-; peno-.

Ex: pen-ile (pertaining to the penis); peni-schisis (a condition in which the penis is fissured); peno-scrotal (pertaining to the penis and the scrotum); peno-genous (originating in the penis); peno-phrenia (preoccupation with thoughts of the penis); peno-phobia (fear of, or aversion for, the penis); peni-form (shaped like a penis).

penis (membrum virile).

(L. *mentula,* penis) mentul-; mentulo-.

Ex: mentul-algia (pain in the penis); mentul-agra (persistent erection); mentulo-mania (abnormal sexual craving for the penis).

penis (symbol of male generative power).

(L. *phallus,* male copulative organ) -phall-; phalli-; phallo-.
Ex: terato-phall-ia (deformity of the penis); phall-itis (inflammation of the penis); phalli-form (having the form of a phallus); phallo-plasty (a plastic operation on the penis); phallic-ism (worship of the phallus as a symbol of generative power); macro-phall-ous (having a large penis).

pepsin.

(Gr. *pepsis,* digestion) pepsin-; pepsini-; pepsino-.
Ex: pepsin-ate (to treat or mix with pepsin); pepsini-ferous (secreting or conveying pepsin); pepsino-genic (producing pepsin).

perception. See under *sensation.*

perforation (puncture; tapping).

(Gr. *kentesis,* puncture) -centesis.
Ex: arthro-centesis (puncture of a joint capsule); abdomino-centesis (puncture of abdominal wall); thoraco-centesis (puncture of chest wall); pericardio-centesis (puncture of the pericardium).

performance. See under *function.*

pericardium.

(Gr. *peri,* surrounding; *kardia,* heart) pericard-; pericardi-; pericardio-.
Ex: paricard-itis (inflammation of the pericardium); pericardi-centesis (surgical puncture of the pericardium); pericardio-pleural (pertaining to the pericardium and the pleura).

perineum.

(Gr. *perineos,* perineum) perine-; perineo-.
Ex: perine-al (pertaining to the perineum); perineo-plasty (a plastic operation on the perineum); perineo-scrotal (pertaining to the perineum and the scrotum).

periosteum.

(Gr. *peri,* surrounding; *osteon,* bone) perioste-; periosteo-; periost-.
Ex: perioste-itis (inflammation of the periosteum); periosteo-

rrhapy (an operation in which a cut or lacerated periosteum is sutured); periost-itis; pesiost-oma (an abnormal growth surrounding the periosteum).

peritoneum.

(L. *peritoneum,* petitoneum) peritone-; peritoneo-; periton-.

Ex: peritone-algia (pain in the peritoneum); peritoneo-centesis (surgical puncture of the peritoneum); peritoneo-pericardial (pertaining to the peritoneum and the pericardium); periton-itis (inflammation of the peritoneum).

personal (one's own; its own; peculiar to the individual; distinct).

(Gr. *idios,* one's own) idio-.

Ex: idio-gamist (male capable of coitus with only one particular female); idio-pathy (primary disease; disease of its own origin); idio-syncrasy; idio-ventricular (pertaining to a ventricle alone).

perspiration. See under *sweat.*

pertaining to.

(Gr.) -ac.

Ex: cardi-ac (pertaining to the heart); ili-ac (pertaining to the ilium).

petrous portion of temporal bone.

(L. *petra,* stone) petro-; petros-.

Ex: petro-mastoid (pertaining to the petrous portion of the temporal bone and the mastoid); petros-ectomy (excision of a part of the petrous portion of the tempral bone); petro-sphenoid.

phalanx (bone of finger or toe).

(L. *phalanx,* line of battle; genit. *phalangis*) -phalang-; pha-lange-; phalangi-; phalango-.

Ex: sym-phalang-ism (fusion of the phalanges); inter-phalange-al (between phalanges); phalangi-form (shaped like a pha-lanx); phalango-phalangeal (pertaining to two adjacent pha-langes); phalang-ectomy (surgical removal of a phalanx).

pharynx (throat).

(Gr. *pharynx,* throat; genit. *pharyngos*) pharyng-; pharyngo-; pharynge-.

Ex: pharyng-ismus (a spasm of the pharynx); pharyng-odynia (pain in the pharynx); pharyngo-nasal (pertaining to the pharynx and the nose); pharyngo-tomy (a surgical cutting into the pharynx); retro-pharynge-al (behind the pharynx).

phenol (carbolic acid).

(Gr. *phainein*, shine) phenol-; phenolo-.

Ex: phenol-ate (to subject to action of phenol); phenol-ic (pertaining to phenol); phenolo-lipoid (a compound of phenol and a lipoid); phenol-phthalein.

phosphate. See under *phosphorus.*

phosphoric acid. See under *phosphorus.*

phosphorus (phosphoric acid; phosphate).

(Gr. *phos*, light; *pherein*, to bear) -phosph-; phospho-; phosphor-; phosphoro-; phosphat-.

Ex: phosph-ate (a salt of phosphoric acid); phospho-protein (a compound of a protein and phosphorus); phosphor-ate (to combine with phosphorus); phosphoro-lysis (the separation of phosphoric acid from a compound); phosphat-emia (an increase in the blood phosphates).

photograh. See under *light.*

phrenic nerve. See under *diaphragm.*

phylum. See under *tribe.*

physical agents. See under *nature.*

physician (medicine; cure; treatment).

(Gr. *iatros*, physician) iatr-; iatro-.

Ex: iatr-aliptic (treatment by inunction); iatro-genic (caused by a physician); iatro-phobia (aversion for, or fear of, physicians).

picture. See under *image* and *paint.*

pigment. See under *color.*

pimple. See under *papule.*

pinworm (threadworm; seatworm; oxyurid).

(Gr. *oxys*, sharp; *oura*, tail) oxyur-; oxyuri-.

Ex: oxyur-iasis (infestation with pinworms); oxyuri-cide (an agent which destroys oxyurids); oxyuri-fuge (an agent which expels pinworms).

pituitary gland (hypophysis).

(L. *pituita*, phlegm) pituitari-; pituit-; pituito-; pituitr-.

Ex: pituitari-genic (caused by the pituitary gland); pituitectomy (the excision of the pituitary gland); pituito-tropic (influenced by the pituitary gland); pituitr-ism (a disorder of the pituitary gland).

place (area; region).

(Gr. *topos,* place) top-; topo-.

Ex: top-*agnosis* (inability to localize touch sensation); top-esthesia (the ability to localize touch sensation); topo-graphy (the description of a region); topo-phobia (fear of a particular place).

placenta.

(L. *placenta,* a cake) placent-; placenti-; placento-.

Ex: placent-ation (the development and attachment of the placenta); placenti-form (shaped like a placenta); placento-pathy (any disorder of the placenta).

plant (vegetable).

(Gr. *phyton,* plant) -phyt-; -phyte; phyto-.

Ex: tricho-phyt-osis (an infection by a fungus); bryo-phyte (a moss or liverwort); phyto-pathology (the study of plant diseases); phyto-plasm (plant protoplasm); phyto-toxin (a toxin produced by a plant).

plasma (protoplasm).

(Gr. *plasma,* formed substance) -plasm-; plasma-; plasmo-.

Ex: proto-plasm-ic (pertaining to protoplasm); plasma-cyte (a plasma cell); plasmo-lysis (lysis of protoplasm); plasmo-schisis (the fragmentation of protoplasm).

plastic surgery (formation; repair).

(Gr. *plastos,* formed) -plasty.

Ex: ano-plasty (a plastic operation on the anus); bleapharo-plasty (a plastic operation on an eyelid); dermato-plasty (a plastic operation on the skin).

plate. See under *squama.*

plate, thin. See under *lamella* and *lamina.*

platelet, blood.

(Gr. *thrombos,* clot; *kytos,* cell) thrombocyt-; thrombocyto-.

Ex: thrombocyto-crit (an instrument to determine the volume of platelets); thrombocyto-lysis (lysis of blood platelets);

thrombocyto-penia (a decrease in the number of blood plate-lets).

pleura (the side).

(Gr. *pleura,* side) pleur-; pleura-; pleuro-.

Ex: pleur-algic (pertaining to pain in the pleura); pleur-ectomy (excision of a part of the pleura); pleuro-centesis (a surgical puncture of the pleura); pleuro-peritoneal (pertaining to the pleura and the peritoneum).

point (dot).

(L. *punctum,* point) punct-; puncti-; puncto-.

Ex: punct-ate (marked by dots or points); puncti-form (resembling a point); puncto-graph (an instrument for localizing foreign bodies).

pointed (sharp).

(Gr. *oxys,* sharp) oxy-.

Ex: oxy-cephaly (a condition in which the top of the cranium is relatively pointed); oxy-urid (a parasitic worm having pointed ends); oxy-rhine (having a pointed nose).

pointed object. See under *needle.*

poison. See under *toxin.*

pollen.

(L. *pollen,* pollen) genit. *pollinis*) pollin-; pollini-.

Ex: pollin-osis (the allergic reaction caused by pollen); pollini-ferous (bearing pollen); pollini-genous (caused by pollen).

pons (pons varolii).

(L. *pons,* a bridge) pont-; ponto-.

Ex: pont-ile (pertaining to the pons); ponto-cerebellar (pertaining to the pons and the cerebellum); sub-pont-ine (below the pons).

poor (poverty).

(Gr. *ptochos,* a beggar) ptoch-; ptochi-; ptocho-.

Ex: ptocho-logy (the study of conditions prevailing among the poor); ptocho-genous (induced by poverty); ptocho-philous (afflicting mainly the poor).

pore. See under *mouth.*

portal vein.

(Gr. *pyle,* gate; *phleps,* vein; genit. *phlebos*) -pyl-; pyle-; pylo-; pylephleb-.

Ex: pyl-ic (pertaining to the portal vein); pyl-emphraxis (obstruction of the portal vein); pylephleb-itis (inflammation of the portal vein); pylephleb-ectasis (abnormal dilatation of the portal vein).

posterior (behind; in the back).

(L. *posterus,* behind) postero-.

Ex: postero-lateral (in the back and to the side); postero-inferior (behind and below); postero-temporal (in the back, or the back part, of the temporal bone).

posterior. See under *back.*

potassium.

(L. *kalium,* potassium) kal-; kali-; kalio-.

Ex: kal-emia (presence of excessive amounts of potassium in the blood); kalio-penia (decrease in the amount of potassium in the body); kali-uresis (elimination of potassium in the urine).

poverty. See under *deficiency* and *poor.*

power (force; strength).

(Gr. *dynamis,* power) dynam-; dynamo-; -dynamous.

Ex: dynam-ic (pertaining to power or force); dynamo-meter (instrument for measuring force, as of muscular contraction); nucleo-dynamous (pertaining to nuclear power).

precipitate. See under *sediment.*

preferring. See under *loving.*

pregnancy (conception).

(Gr. *kyesis,* gestation) cyes-; cyesi-; cyeso-; cyesio-.

Ex: cyes-edema (swelling observed in pregnant women); cyesio-logy (the science of pregnancy).

pregnant (pregnancy).

(L. *gravida,* heavy) gravid-; gravido-; -gravida.

Ex: gravid-ism (the condition of being pregnant); gravid-ity (pregnancy); multi-gravida (a woman who has borne several children).

preservation. See under *protection.*

pressure.

(Gr. *piezein,* to press; *piesis,* pressure) pies-; piesi-; pieso-; piez-; piezo-.

Ex: pies-esthesia (the sensation or perception of pressure); piesi-meter (an instrument to measure sensitiveness to pressure); piezo-therapy (the use of pressure in treatment, as in pneumothorax).

pressure.

(L. *pressura,* pressure) presso-; pressur-; pressuro-.

Ex: presso-meter (an instrument used to measure pressure); presso-receptive (activated by stimuli due to pressure); pressuro-genous (caused by pressure). See also *weight.*

pretended. See under *false.*

primitive (original; first in time; beginning).

(Gr. *arche*) arch-; arche-; archi-.

Ex: arch-encephalon (primitive brain); arche-gonium; arche-type (original type); archi-plasm (primitive living matter).

primitive. See under *earliest* and *old.*

primordium. See under *sprout.*

prior. See under *before.*

prism (prismatic lens).

(L. *prisma,* prism) prism-; prismat-; prismato-.

Ex: prism-oid (shaped like a prism); prismat-ic (pertaining to, or produced by, a prism); prismato-meter (an instrument for measuring prisms).

process (formation; cause of action; abnormal condition).

(Gr.) -iasis.

Ex: cholelith-iasis (process of formation of gallstones); mydr-iasis (abnormal dilatation of pupil); odont-iasis (the process of eruption or appearance of the teeth).

produce (beget; cause; originate).

(L. *generare,* beget) gener-; -gener-.

Ex: gener-ate (produce or beget); con-gener-ous (allied in origin).

producer (something that produces).

(L. genesis, origin) -gen.

Ex: patho-gen (microorganism causing disease); aller-gen

(something producing an allergic reaction); pyro-gen (something producing fever).

production (formation; making).

(Gr. *poiesis,* a making) -poiesis; -poietic.

Ex: hemato-poiesis (formation of blood); chole-poiesis (formation of bile); galacto-poietic (producing milk).

projection, rounded. See under *condyle.*

prostate gland.

(Gr. *prostates,* something standing before) prostat-; prostatico-; prostato-.

Ex: prostat-ectomy (excision of the prostate); prostatico-vesical (pertaining to the prostate and the bladder); prostato-vesiculitis (inflammation of the prostate and the seminal vesicles).

prosthesis (artificial structure).

(Gr. *prosthesis,* an addition) prosth-; prosthet-; prostho-.

Ex: prosth-odontics (dentistry dealing with artificial teeth and parts); prosth-odontist; prosthet-ics (the science and art of replacing missing body parts by artificial structures).

prostitute (harlot).

(Gr. *porne,* harlot) porne-; porno-.

Ex: porno-lagnia (a keen sexual desire for prostitutes); porno-phobia (fear of prostitutes); porno-logy (study of prostitutes and prostitution); porno-therapy (medical control and treatment of prostitutes).

protection (defense; preservation).

(Gr. *phylassein,* to defend; *phylaktikos,* guarding) -phylact-; phylacto-.

Ex: pro-phylact-ic (guarding against a disease); phylact-ic (protecting); phylacto-genic (producing a defense against a disease); phylacto-lytic (destroying the protection against a disease).

protein.

(Gr. *proteios,* prime) protein-; proteino-; proteo-.

Ex: protein-ase (an enzyme aiding in the digestion of proteins); proteino-genous (originating from protein); proteo-lytic (pertaining to the lysis of proteins).

protoplasm. See under *plasma.*

provoking. See under *stimulating.*

psyche. See under *mind.*

pterygoid process. See under *wing.*

puberty.

(L. *pubertas,* of ripe age) puber-; pubert-; puberto-.

Ex: puber-al (pertaining to the age of puberty); pubert-al (characteristic of puberty); puberto-philous (fond of puberty) occurring mainly at puberty); puberto-trichia (the growth of hair characteristic of puberty).

pubic bone.

(L. *pubis,* pubic bone) pub-; pubio-; pubo-.

Ex: pub-ic (pertaining to the pubic bone); pubio-tomy (the surgical cutting of the juncture between the two pubic bones); pubo-vesical (pertaining to the pubic bones and the bladder).

pulp (dental pulp).

(L. *pulpa,* flesh) pulp-; pulpi-; pulpo-.

Ex: pulp-algia (pain in the pulp of a tooth); pulp-ectomy (surgical removal of the pulp from a tooth); pulp-itis; pulpo-lingual (pertaining to the pulpal wall and lingual wall of a tooth cavity).

pulse.

(Gr. *sphygmos,* pulse) sphygmo-.

Ex: sphygmo-gram (a tracing depicting the movements of the pulse); sphygmo-meter (an instrument used to measure the pulse); sphygmo-cardiograph (an instrument for recording the pulse and the heart beat).

puncture. See under *perforation.*

punishment (discipline; chastisement).

(L. *poena,* punishment) -pen-; pena-; peno-.

Ex: philo-pen-ia (an abnormal desire to be punished); pena-genous (derived from punishment); peno-logy (the study of punishment); peno-phobia (fear of punishment).

pupil of eye.

(Gr. *kore,* pupil) cor-; cori-; coro-; core-; coreo-.

Ex: cor-ectasis (dilatation of the pupil); cor-ectopia (displacement of the pupil); diplo-cor-ia (condition of having a double

pupil); core-clisis (abnormal closure of a pupil); coreo-me-
ter (an instrument for measuring the pupil); coro-tomy (incision of the iris near the pupil).

pupil of eye.

(L. *pupilla*, pupil) pupill-; pupillo-.

Ex: pupill-atonia (a condition in which the pupil does not
react to light); pupillo-meter (an instrument used to measure
the size of the pupil); pupillo-motor (pertaining to the contraction and dilatation of the pupil).

pus.

(L. *pus*, pus; genit. *puris*) -pur-; puri-.

Ex: sup-pur-ation (the formation of pus); puri-form (resembling pus); pur-ulent (containing, or marked by the formation of, pus).

pus.

(Gr. *pyon*, pus) -py-; pyo-.

Ex: em-py-ema (an accumulation of pus in the pleural cavity);
py-uria (presence of pus in the urine); pyo-derma (a skin
disease marked by the formation of pus); pyo-hemothorax (the
presence of pus and blood in the pleural cavity).

pustule.

(L. *pustula*, pustule) pustul-; pustuli-; pustulo-.

Ex: pustul-ant (an agent which causes the formation of pustules); pustul-ation (the formation of pustules); pustuli-form
(having the form of a pustule); pustulo-papular (marked by
the presence of both pustules and papules).

putrefaction (decomposition).

(Gr. *septos*, putrid) sept-; septic-; septico-.

Ex: septi-genic (causing putrefaction); septic-emia (the presence of bacterial products in the blood); septico-pyemia (a
condition marked by septicemia and pyemia).

putrefying. See under *decaying*.

pylorus.

(Gr. *pyloros*, pylorus; *pyle*, gate) pylor-; pyloro-.

Ex: pylor-ectomy (the surgical excision of the pylorus);
pyloro-plasty (a plastic operation on the pylorus); pyloro-
spasm (a spastic contraction of the pylorus).

pyrexia. See under *fever*.

Q

quarter (one fourth).

(L. *quadrans,* quarter; genit *quadrantis*) quadrant-; quadranto-

Ex: quadrant-al (pertaining to a quadrant or quarter of a circle); quadrant-anopia (defective vision in one fourth of the visual field).

quiescent. See under *sleep.*

quiver. See under *vibration.*

R

rabies (hydrophobia).

(Gr. *lyssa,* frenzy) lysso-.

Ex: lysso-dexis (bite of a rabid animal); lysso-phobia (fear of rabies).

rabies (hydrophobia).

(L. *rabies,* madness) rab-; rabi-.

Ex: rab-id (affected by rabies); rabi-form (resembling rabies); rabi-phylactic (preventing rabies); rabi-genic (causing rabies); rabi-genous (caused by rabies).

race (kind; sex).

(Gr. *genos,* race) geno-.

Ex: geno-type (typical species of a genus); geno-me (set of hereditary factors); geno-phobia (fear of sexual relations).

radiation (radiant energy; radium).

(L. *radius,* ray) radio-.

Ex: radio-activity (the process of giving off radiant energy); radio-biology (the study of the effect of radiation on living organisms); radio-carbon (a radioactive isotope of carbon); radio-curable (curable by radiation).

radium. See under radiation.

radius.

(L. *radius,* a rod) radi-; radio-.

Ex: radi-al (pertaining to the radius); radio-carpal (pertaining to the radius and the carpus); radio-ulnar (pertaining to the radius and the ulna).

ramus. See under *branch.*

rapid (fast; swift).

(Gr. *tachys,* swift) tacho-; tachy-.

Ex: tacho-meter (a device used to measure the speed of the blood flow); tachy-cardia; tachy-phagia (rapid eating); tachy-pnea (rapid breathing).

ray (beam).

(Gr. *aktis,* ray; genit. *aktinos*) actin-; actini-; actino-.

Ex: actin-ic (pertaining to rays); actini-form (resembling a ray or rays); actin-ism (the functional property of radiant energy); actino-genesis (production of rays); Actino-myces (a genus of microorganisms occurring in formations resembling rays).

receive (take; accept).

(L. *receptus,* received) cept-; cepti-; cepto-.

Ex: extero-cepti-ve (receiving stimuli from external environment); extero-cept-or (nerve receiving stimuli from external environment); noci-cept-or (nerve receiving stimuli caused by injury).

recent. See under *new.*

recognition. See under *knowledge.*

record. See under *write.*

recording. See under *tracing.*

rectum (anus).

(Gr. *archos,* rectum) archo-.

Ex: archo-cele (hernia of the rectum); archo-rrhagia (bleeding from the rectum); archo-stenosis.

rectum (anus).

(Gr. *proktos,* anus) proct-; procto-.

Ex: proct-ectasia (an abnormal dilatation of the rectum); proct-itis (inflammation of the rectum); procto-logy (the branch of medicine dealing with the rectum); procto-plasty (a plastic operation on the rectum and anus).

rectum (intestinum rectum).

(L. *rectum,* straight) rect-; recto-.

Ex: rect-algia (pain in the rectum); recto-cele (herniation of a part of the rectum); recto-sigmoid (pertaining to the rectum and the sigmoid); recto-vaginal (pertaining to the rectum and the vagina).

red (reddening; reddish).

(L. *ruber,* red; *rubricatus,* reddened; *rubefacere,* to redden) rube-; rubi-; rubid-; rubri-; rubro-.

Ex: rube-facient (an agent which reddens the skin); rube-osis (abnormal reddening of the skin); rubid-ium; rubri-cyte (a kind of erythroblast); rubro-spinal (pertaining to the red nucleus and the spine).

red (reddish).

(Gr. *erythros,* red) erysi-; eryth-; erythr-; erythro-.

Ex: erysi-pelas (red skin; skin disease marked by redness, etc.); erythr-algia (redness of the skin); erythro-cyte (red blood cell).

red See under *rose.*

reflex (reflex action).

(L. *reflectere,* to reflect; pp. *reflexus*) -reflex-; reflexo-; reflexi-.
Ex: a-reflex-ia (absence of reflexes); hyper-reflex-ia (condition of having hyperactive reflexes); reflexo-genic (producing a reflex; intensifying reflex action); reflexo-therapy (treatment based on the principle of reflex action); reflexi-motor (pertaining to motor part of a reflex action).

refraction.

(L. *refringere,* to break; pp. *refractus*) refract-; refracto-; refrang-.

Ex: refract-ive (capable of refracting); refracto-meter (an instrument for measuring refraction); refracto-metry; refrangible (capable of being refracted).

region. See under *place.*

religion (sacredness).

(Gr. *hieros,* sacred) hier-; hiero-.

Ex: hiero-mania (a mania about a religious matter or sacred thing); hiero-therapy (treatment of disease by religious faith or rites).

remembrance. See under *memory.*

remote. See under *distal.*

repair. See under *plastic surgery.*

repetition. See under *again* and *imitation.*

reproduction (sexual organs; birth).

(L. *genere,* beget; *genitalis,* genital) genit-; genital-; genito-.
Ex: genit-alia (reproductive organs); genito-femoral (pertaining to the genital organs and the thigh); genito-urinary (pertaining to the reproductive organs and the urinary system).

reproductive cell. See under *gamete* and *spore.*

resembling (like; having the form of).

(Gr. *eidos,* form; *oeides,* in the form of) eid-; eido-; -ode; -oid; -oidal; -oidea; -oidus.

Ex: nemat-ode (a worm resembling a thread); nemat-oid (resembling a thread); Echin-oidea (the sea urchins); rhomb-oideus (a muscle having the form of a rhomboid or rhombus).

resilient. See under *elastic.*

resistance. See under *immunity.*

respiration (breathing).

(L. *respirare,* to breathe; pp. *respiratus*) respir-; respirat-; respiro-.

Ex: respir-able (that may be respired); respir-ation; respirat-or (an apparatus for administering artificial respiration); respiro-meter (an instrument used to measure the respiratory movements).

respiration. See under *air* and *breathe.*

rete (net; network).

(L. *rete,* a net; pl. *retia*) ret-; reti-.

Ex: reti-al (pertaining to a rete); reti-form (having the form of a net); reti-ation (the formation of a network).

reticulocyte.

(L. *reticulum,* a small net; Gr. *kytos,* a cell) reticulocyt-; reticulocyto-.

Ex: reticulocyt-osis (an abnormal condition marked by an increase in the number of reticulocytes); reticulocyto-genic (producing reticulocytes); reticulocyto-penia (an abnormal decrease in the number of reticulocytes).

reticulum (network; net).

(L. *reticulum,* a small net) reticul-; reticulo-.

Ex: reticul-ar (resembling a net); reticulo-cyte (a young red blood cell having a reticulum); reticulo-endothelial (pertaining to reticular and endothelial tissues).

retina.

(L. *rete,* a net; genit. *retis*) retin-; retino-.

Ex: retin-itis (inflammation of the retina); retino-choroid (the retina and the choroid as a single structure); retino-pathy (any disease of the retina).

reversal. See under *other.*

rheumatism.

(Gr. *rheuma,* discharge) rheumat-; rheumato-.

Ex: rheumat-algia (rheumatic pain); rheumat-ismal (pertaining to rheumatism); rheumat-oid (resembling rheumatism); rheumato-genic (causing rheumatism).

rhythm.

(Gr. *rhythmos,* rhythm-; rrhythm-; rhythmo-.

Ex: a-rrhythm-ia (lack of normal rhythm); eu-rhythm-ia (normal rhythm); rhythm-icity (the condition of being rhythmical); rhythmo-therapy (treatment by the use of rhythm).

rib (rib-like ridge).

(L. *costa,* rib) cost-; costi-; costo-.

Ex: cost-algia (pain in a rib); costi-cartilage (cartilage of a rib); costo-clavicular (pertaining to a rib and a clavicle).

rickettsia.

(Howard T. *Ricketts*) ricketts-; rickettsi-; rickettsio-.

Ex: ricketts-emia (presence of rickettsiae in the blood stream); rickettsi-al (pertaining to rickettsiae); rickettsi-cidal (capable of killing rickettsiae); rickettsio-genous (caused by rickettsiae).

ridge. See under *crest* and *fold.*

right (right side).

(L. *dexter,* right) dextr-; dextri-; dextro-.

Ex: dextr-aural (hearing better with the right ear); dextro-cardia (condition of having the heart on the right side); dextro-rotatory (capable of turning the plane of polarized light to the right); ambi-dextr-ous (equally skilled or facile with both hands).

rind. See under *cortex.*

rocky. See under *hard.*

rod-like structure. See under *striated muscle fiber.*

roentgen (x-rays).

(Wilhelm K. *Roentgen*) roetgen-; roentgeno-.

Ex: roentgen-ize (to subject to the action of roentgen rays); roentgeno-gram (a picture produced by the action of roentgen rays); roentgeno-logy; roentgen-opaque (opaque to x-rays).

roof of mouth. See under *palate.*

root.

(L. *radix,* root) radici-; radico-; radicul-; radiculo-.

Ex: radici-form (resembling a root); radico-tomy (the surgical cutting of a root); radicul-ectomy (excision of a root); radiculo-medullary (pertaining to nerve roots and the spinal cord).

root (spinal nerve root).

(Gr. *rhiza,* root) rhiz-; rhizo-.

Ex: rhiz-ectomy (excision of a root); rhizo-tomy (the surgical cutting of a root); rhizo-genic (producing roots); rhizo-morphous (resembling a root).

rose (rose-red; red).

(Gr. *rhodon,* rose) rhod-; rhodo-.

Ex: rhod-amine (a pink dye); Rhodo-coccus (microorganism producing a red pigment); rhod-opsin (visual purple); rhodo-phylactic (restoring visual purple).

rot. See under *decay.*

rotation (twisting; turning).

(L. *torquere,* twist; *tortus,* twisted) torsi-; torsio-; torso-; torti-. *Ex*: torsio-meter (an instrument for measuring rotation); torso-occlusion (rotation of a tooth); torti-collis (wryneck). See also *circle.*

round (spherical; sphere).

(Gr. *sphaira,* ball) sphero-.

Ex: sphero-cyte (a spherical red blood cell); sphero-lith (a spherical renal calculus); sphero-plast (a spherical cell).

roundworm. See under *earthworm.*

rubbing (grinding; friction).

(Gr. *tripsis,* a rubbing) -tripsis.

Ex: hemocyto-tripsis (a fragmentation of red blood cells

caused by friction or grinding); odonto-tripsis (a wearing away of tooth substance by friction); dermato-tripsis (an abrasion of skin by rubbing or friction).

rump. See under *buttock.*

running (conduction; race course).

(Gr. *dromos,* race course) drom-; dromi-; dromo-.

Ex: dromo-mania (a compulsion to roam or move from place to place); dromo-tropic (affecting the conducting quality of a nerve fiber); dromo-meter (instrument to measure speed); pro-drom-al (coming before; premonitory).

rupture. See under *break.*

S

sac (pouch).

(L. *saccus,* sac) sacc-; sacci-; saccul-.

Ex: sacc-ate (shaped like, or containing, a sac); sacci-form (having the shape of a sac); saccul-ar (of the nature of a sac); saccul-ation (the condition of having sacs or a sac). See also *bladder,* and *follicle.*

sacred. See under *religion.*

sacrum.

(L. *sacrum,* sacred) sacr-; sacro-.

Ex: sacr-al (pertaining to the sacrum); sacr-algia (pain in the sacrum); sacro-spinal (pertaining to the sacrum and the spine); sacro-iliac (pertaining to the sacrum and the ilium).

sagging. See under *drooping.*

saliva.

(Gr. *sialon,* saliva) sial-; sialo-.

Ex: sialo-genic (producing saliva); sialo-lithiasis (the forma-tion or presence of salivary calculi); sialo-rrhea (excessive flow of saliva).

saliva (spittle).

(Gr. *ptyalon,* spittle) ptyal-; ptyalo-.

Ex: ptyal-agogue (a substance which stimulates the formation of saliva); ptyal-ism (excessive formation of saliva); ptyalo-reaction (a chemical reaction caused by or in saliva).

salivary gland.
 (Gr. *sialon,* saliva; *aden,* gland) sialoaden-; sialoadeno-.
 Ex: sialoaden-itis (inflammation of a salivary gland); sialoa-deno-tomy (surgical incision into a salivary gland).

same (sameness; similarity; unchanging condition).
 (Gr. *homoios,* like; *homos,* same) hemeo-; homoio-; homo-.
 Ex: homeo-morphous (similar or like in form); homeo-plasia (growth of new tissue which is similar to adjacent tissue); homoio-thermy (the condition of having an unchanging body temperature); homo-geneous (having a uniform consistency throughout).

same (self; one's own).
 (Gr. *ipsos,* same; L. *ipse,* self) ips-; ipsi-.
 Ex: ips-ation (self-gratification); ipsi-lateral (pertaining to the same side).

same (the same).
 (Gr. *to auto,* the same) tauto-.
 Ex: tauto-menial (involving the same menstrual period); tauto-merism; tauto-logy (repetition of words); tauto-phony (repetition of the same sound). See also *equal.*

same time. See under *with.*

scale (flake; husk).
 (Gr. *lepis,* scale; genit. *lepidos; lepos,* scale) lepid-; lepido-; lepo-.
 Ex: lepid-ic (pertaining to, or covered with, scales); lepid-osis (a skin disorder marked by scaling); lepo-thrix (a disorder of hair marked by scaliness).

scale. See under *lamella* and *squama.*

scanty. See under *few.*

scapula (shoulder blade).
 (L. *scapula,* shoulder) scapul-; scapulo-.
 Ex: scapul-ar (pertaining to the scapula); scapul-ectomy (surgical removal of the scapula or a part thereof); scapulo-clavicular (pertaining to the scapula and the clavicle).

scar (scar tissue).
 (Gr. *oule,* scar) ul-. uli-; ulo-.
 Ex: ul-ectomy (excision of a scar); uli-form (resembling a

scar); ulo-tomy (the cutting of scar tissue); ulo-genous (arising in scar tissue).

scar (cicatrix; new tissue).

(L. *cicatrix,* scar) cicatr-; cicatrici-; cicatrico-; cicatri-.

Ex: cicatr-ectomy (excision of a scar); cicatrici-al (pertaining to a scar); cicatrix; cicatri-zation (healing associated with scar formation).

scarcity (fewness).

(Gr. *spanos,* scarce) span-; spano-.

Ex: span-emia (a scarcity of the formed elements in the blood); spano-gyny (scarcity of females); spano-menorrhea (infrequent or scanty menstruation).

scarcity. See under *deficiency.*

science of (study of; branch of knowledge).

(Gr. *logos,* study) -logy.

Ex: bio-logy; physio-logy; endocrino-logy (the science or study of endocrine glands); onco-logy (the study of tumors); dermato-logy.

sclera.

(Gr. *skleros,* hard) scler-; sclero-.

Ex: scler-ectomy (excision of a portion of the sclera); scler-itis (inflammation of the sclera); sclero-choroiditis (inflammation of the sclera and the choroid); sclero-corneal (pertaining to the sclera and the cornea).

sclerous. See under *hard.*

scotoma. See under *darkness.*

scrotum.

(Gr. *oscheon,* scrotum) osche-; oscheo-.

Ex: osche-itis (inflammation of the scrotum); osche-algia (pain in the scrotum); osche-oma (a tumor of the scrotum); oscheo-plasty (a plastic operation on the scrotum).

scrotum.

(L. *scrotum,* bag) scrot-; scroto-.

Ex: scrot-al (pertaining to the scrotum); scrot-ectomy (excision of a part or all of the scrotum); scrot-itis (inflammation of the scrotum); scroto-plasty (a plastic operation on the scrotum).

seatworm. See under *pinworm.*

sebum (fatty secretion).

(L. *sebum,* tallow) seb-; sebi-; sebo-.

Ex: seb-aceous (of the nature of sebum); sebi-ferous (producing or bearing sebum); sebo-rrhea; sebo-rrheal (marked by a discharge of sebum).

second (following another).

(L. *secundus,* second) secundi-; secundo-.

Ex: secundi-gravida (a woman who is pregnant for the second time); secundi-para (a woman who had two childbirths); secundo-geniture (the condition or status of being born second).

second (secondary).

(Gr. *deuteros,* second) deuter-; deutero-; deuto-.

Ex: deuter-anopia (a defect or color vision marked by ability to perceive only two colors); deutero-pathy (a secondary disease); deuto-plasm (passive or secondary materials in the protoplasm of a cell, or yolk).

secret. See under *hidden.*

secretion.

(L. *secernere,* to separate; pp. *secretus*) secret-; secreto-.

Ex: secret-in (a hormone produced in the duodenum and jejunum); secreto-dermatosis (an abnormality of the secreting functions of the skin); secreto-motor (serving to stimulate secretion).

secretion (elaboration).

(Gr. *krinein,* to separate) crin-; crino-.

Ex: crino-genic (producing a secretion); endo-crino-logy (science of internal secretions).

section (a cutting).

(L. *secare,* to cut; pp. *sectus*) -sect-; -section; sectori-.

Ex: sect-ile (capable of being cut); hemi-section (a section along the midline); sectori-al (adapted for cutting).

securing. See under *fixation.*

security. See under *immunity.*

sediment (sedimentation; precipitate).

(L. *sedimentum,* a sediment) sediment-; sedimenti-; sedimento-.

Ex: sediment-ation (the formation of a sediment); sediment-ary (pertaining to a sediment); sedimenti-form (resembling a sediment); sedimento-genic (promoting the formation of a sediment).

seed. See under *semen* and *spermatozoa.*

seeking. See under *moving toward.*

segment. See under *part.*

self (oneself; own).

(Gr. *autos,* self) aut-; auto-.

Ex: auto-analysis (analysis of oneself); auto-didact (a self-taught person); auto-erotism; auto-hemolysis.

self. See under *same.*

semen.

(L. *semen,* a seed; genit. *seminis*) semi-; semini-; semino-.

Ex: semin-ation (introduction of semen); semini-ferous (conveying semen); semino-logy (the study of semen).

semen (sperm; seed).

(Gr. *gone,* seed) gon-; gone-; gono-.

Ex: gone-cyst (a seminal vesicle); gone-poiesis (formation of semen); gono-cyte (primitive reproductive cell).

semilunar. See under *sickle.*

seminal vesicle.

(Gr. *gone,* seed; *kystis,* bladder) gonecyst-; gonecysto-.

Ex: gonecyst-itis (inflammation of a seminal vesicle); gonecysto-lith (a calculus in a seminal vesicle); gonecyst-ectomy (excision of a seminal vesicle); gonecyst-algia (pain in a seminal vesicle).

sensation (feeling; perception).

(L. *aesthesia,* perception) esthes-; esthesi-; esthesio-; esthet-.

Ex: esthes-ia (feeling); an-esthet-ic (without sensation); esthesio-meter (instrument for measuring tactile sensation).

sensation (sensory; sense).

(L. *sensus,* sense) sens-; sensi-; senso-; sensori-.

Ex: sensi-ferous (conveying sensory impulses); sensi-meter (an instrument used to measure sensitiveness); senso-motor (pertaining to sensory and motor functions); sensori-muscular (pertaining to muscular and sensory activity).

sensitive. See under *sharp.*

separation (reversal).

   (L.) di-; dis-.

   Ex: dis-infection (separation from infection); dis-location (separation from normal location); dis-section (separation by cutting).

separation from. See under *without.*

septum (wall; partition).

   (L. *septum,* hedge) sept-; septo-.

   Ex: sept-al (pertaining to a septum); sept-ation (division by a septum or septa); sept-ectomy (excision of a septum); septo-meter (an instrument used to measure a septum); septo-tomy (a surgical incision into a septum).

serpent. See under *snake.*

serum.

   (L. *serum,* whey) sero-.

   Ex: sero-negative (indicating a negative result based on a test of a given serum); sero-reaction (a reaction in a serum); sero-toxin (a toxin formed in serum).

serum (blood serum).

   (Gr. *orrhos,* serum) orrho-.

   Ex: orrho-diagnosis (diagnosis based on the examination of serum); orrho-logy (serology); orrho-therapy (treatment of disease with serums).

set in motion. See under *excite.*

seven.

   (Gr. *hepta,* seven) hept-; hepta-.

   Ex: hepta-dactylia (the condition of having seven fingers or toes on one limb); hepta-valent (having a chemical valence of seven).

seven (seventh).

   (L. septem, seven) sept-; septa-; septi-.

   Ex: septi-gravida (a woman pregnant for the seventh time); septi-valent (having a valence of seven); septi-para (a woman who has borne seven or more offspring in seven pregnancies).

several (many; more).

(L. *plus,* more; genit. *pluris*) pluri-.

Ex: pluri-glandular (pertaining to several glands); pluri-nuclear (having several nuclei); pluri-resistant (resistant to several drugs, stains).

several. See under *many.*

sewing together. See under *suturing.*

sexual desire (libido; lust).

(L. *libido,* pleasure) libid-; libidin-; libido-.

Ex: libido-genous (motivated by the libido); libido-genic (stimulating sexual desire); libid-agnosia (unawareness of the influence of the libido upon one's actions).

sexual desire (love; sexual love).

(Gr. *eros,* love; *erotikos,* erotic) erot-; eroti-; erotic-; erotico-; eroto-.

Ex: erotic-ism (excessive sexual desire); eroto-genic (stimulating sexual desire); eroto-phobia (aversion for sexual love).

sexual desire. See under *venereal disese.*

sexual organs. See under *reproduction.*

shape. See under *form.*

sharp (keen; acute; sensitive).

(Gr. *oxys,* keen) oxy-.

Ex: oxy-blepsia (unusual sharpness of vision); oxy-geusia (unusual sharpness of the sense of taste); oxy-cusis (unusual sharpness of the sense of hearing); oxy-aphia (a keen sense of touch).

sharp. See under *pointed.*

sheath (case).

(Gr. *theke,* sheath) thec-; theco-.

Ex: thec-al (pertaining to a sheath); thec-itis (inflammation of a tendon sheath); theco-stegnosis (narrowing of a tendon sheath).

shin. See under *leg.*

short (shortness).

(Gr. *brachys,* short) brachy-.

Ex: brachy-cephalic (having a short head); brachy-gnathia (shortness of the jaw); brachy-phalangia.

shoulder.
(Gr. *omos,* shoulder) om-; oma-; omo-.
Ex: om-algia (pain in the shoulder); omo-clavicular (pertaining to, or involving, a shoulder and a clavicle); omo-hyoid (pertaining to a shoulder and the hyoid bone).

shoulder blade. See under *scapula.*

shoulder joint.
(Gr. *omos,* shoulder; *arthron* joint) omarthr-; omarthro-.
Ex: omarthr-itis (inflammation of the shoulder joint); omarthropathy (any disease of the shoulder joint); omarthro-tomy (an incision into the shoulder joint).

sickle (crescent; semilunar).
(Gr. *drepanon,* a sickle) drepan-; drepani-; drepano-.
Ex: drepani-form (shaped like a sickle); drepano-cyte (a red blood cell shaped like a sickle); Drepano-spira (genus of microorganisms).

side (sideways).
(L. *latus,* side; genit. *lateris*) later-; latero-.
Ex: later-ad (toward the side); latero-flexion (flexion to the side); latero-version (a turning to the side).

sight (vision).
(Gr. *blepsis,* sight) -bleps-; blepsia; -blepsy.
Ex: a-blepsia (lack of sight); a-blepsy; mono-blepsia (lack of vision in one eye).

sight. See under *vision* and *optics.*

sigmoid flexure.
(Gr. *sigmoeides,* shaped like the letter S) sigmoid-; sigmoido-.
Ex: sigmoid-ectomy (excision of the sigmoid flexure); sigmoid-itis; sigmoido-scope (an endoscope used in examining the sigmoid); sigmoido-stomy (the formation of a surgical opening in the sigmoid flexure).

silica (silicon).
(L. *silex,* flint; genit. *silicis*) silic-; silico-; silici-.
Ex: silic-ate (a compound or salt of silicic acid); silice-ous (containing silica); silic-osis (a form of pneumoconiosis caused by dust of stone); silico-manganese (an alloy of silicon and manganese).

similar. See under *equal.*

similarity. See under *same.*

simple (single).

(Gr. *haploos,* simple) hapl-; haplo-.

Ex: haplo-dermatitis (simple or uncomplicated dermatitis); hapl-oid (having a single set of chromosomes); haplo-dont (pertaining to a molar tooth without a cusp).

single. See under *one* and *simple.*

sinus.

(L. *sinus,* a fold) sinus-; sinuso-.

Ex: sinus-itis (inflammation of a sinus); sinus-oid (like a sinus); sinuso-tomy (an incision into a sinus); sinuso-logy (the study of sinuses). See also *antrum.*

six

(L. *sex,* six) sex-; sexi-.

Ex: sex-digitate (having six digits); sex-cuspidate (having six cusps); sex-angular (having six angles); sexi-valent (having a valence of six).

six. (sixfold).

(Gr. *hex,* six) hex-; hexa-.

Ex: hex-ose (a sugar containing six carbon atoms); hex-atomic (containing six atoms); hexa-valent (having a chemical valence of six); hexa-dactylia (the condition of having six fingers or six toes on one limb).

sixth.

(L. *sextus,* sixth) sexti-; sextu-.

Ex: sexti-gravida (a woman pregnant for the sixth time); sexti-para (a woman who has borne children in six pregnancies); sextu-plet (one of six children produced in one pregnancy).

skin (dermis; derma).

(Gr. *derma,* skin; genit. *dermatos*) derm-; -derm; derma-; dermo-; dermat-; dermato-.

Ex: derm-al (pertaining to the skin); pachy-derma (thickening of the skin); derma-tome (instrument for cutting thin layers of skin); dermo-mycosis (skin disease caused by fungi); dermat-itis; dermato-logy (science of the skin).

skin (epidermis; membrane).

(L. *cutis,* skin) cut-; cuti-; cuticul-.

Ex: cut-aneous (pertaining to, or composed of, skin); cuti-color (having the color of skin); cuti-reaction (an inflammatory reaction of the skin).

skull. See under *cranium.*

sleep.

(L. *somnus,* sleep) somn-; somni-; somno-.

Ex: somn-ambulism (sleep walking); somni-facient (inducing sleep); somni-loquism (the phenomenon of talking in one's sleep); somno-lism (a hypnotic trance).

sleep (hypnotism).

(Gr. *hypnos,* sleep) hypn-; hypno-.

Ex: hypn-agogue (a substance inducing sleep); hypno-analysis (psychoanalysis performed while the patient is under hypnosis); hypno-genic (producing sleep); hypno-therapy (the application of hypnosis in the treatment of disease).

sleep (sleeping; inactive; quiescent).

(L. *dormire,* sleep) dorm-; dormi-; dormo-.

Ex: dorm-ant (inactive); dormi-facient (inducing sleep); ob-dormi-tion (numbness resulting from pressure on a nerve). See also *stupor.*

sleep, deep.

(L. *sopor,* deep sleep) sopor-; sopori-.

Ex: sopor-ous (marked by deep sleep); sopori-fic (a substance causing profound sleep); sopori-fugic (counteracting profound sleep).

slender (delicate; thin; narrow).

(Gr. *leptos,* slender) lept-; lepto-.

Ex: lepto-dactylous (having slender fingers or toes); lepto-dermic (having a thin skin); lepto-pellic (having a narrow pelvis); lepto-somatic (having a delicate, thin body).

slenderness. See under *spider.*

slow (dull).

(Gr. *bradys,* slow) brady-.

Ex: brady-acusia (dullness of hearing); brady-kinesia (slowness of movement); brady-lexia (slowness in reading).

small (microscopic; one-millionth).

(Gr. *mikros,* small) micr-; micro-.

Ex: micr-encephaly (pathologic smallness of the brain); micro-scope; micro-analysis (analysis of very small quantities of a material); micro-biology; hyper-micro-somia (abnormal smallness of the body); micro-millimeter (one millionth part of a millimeter).

smallness (dwarfishness).

(L. *nanus,* dwarf) nan-; nani-; nano-.

Ex: nani-virus (a kind of very small virus); nano-cephalia (abnormal smallness of the head); nano-melous (having abnormally small limbs).

smallpox.

(L. *variola,* smallpox) variol-; varioli-; variolo-.

Ex: variol-ation (inoculation with smallpox virus); varioliform (resembling smallpox); variolo-vaccine (smallpox vaccine).

smell (odor).

(Gr. *osme,* smell) osm-; osmio-; osmo-.

Ex: osm-esthesia (perception of odors); osmo-lagnia (sexual desire stimulated by certain odors); osmo-phobia (an aversion for certain odors).

smell (sense of smell).

(Gr. *osphresis,* sense of smell) -osphresia; osphresio-.

Ex: oxy-osphresia (sharpness of the sense of smell); osphresiology (the study of the sense of smell and odors); osphresio-lagnic (a person who is readily stimulated sexually by certain odors).

smell (sense of smell; act of smelling).

(L. *olfacere,* to smell; pp. *olfactus*) olfact-; olfacti-; olfacto-.

Ex: olfact-ion (the act of smelling); olfacto-meter (an instrument for testing the sense of smell); olfacto-phobia (an aversion for smelling certain odors).

smooth (unwrinkled; glossy).

(Gr. *leios,* smooth) leio-.

Ex: leio-dermia (smoothness of the skin); leio-myoma (a tumor of smooth muscle). See also *even.*

snake (serpent).

> (Gr. *ophidion,* serpent; *ophis,* snake) ophid-; ophidio-.
>
> *Ex*: ophid-ic (pertaining to snakes); ophidio-phobia (excessive fear of snakes); ophio-toxemia (the toxemia resulting from snake venom).

soap.

> (L. *sapo,* soap; genit. *saponis*) sapo-; sapon-; saponi-.
>
> *Ex*: sapo-genic (forming soap); sapon-aceous (having the quality of soap); saponi-fication (a chemical process in which soap is formed).

socket. See under *alveolus.*

soft (abnormal softness).

> (Gr. *malakos,* soft) malac-; malaco-.
>
> *Ex*: malac-ia (abnormal softness of a structure); malaco-plakia (presence of soft patches).

soft palate. See under *palate.*

soil. See under *earth.*

solid (three-dimensional).

> (Gr. *stereos,* solid) stereo-.
>
> *Ex*: stereo-arthrolysis (surgical formation of a new joint); stereo-gnosis (the perception of the form of objects by touch); stereo-scope (an instrument which gives a three-dimensional appearance to flat pictures). See also *thick.*

solution (dissolving).

> (Gr. *lyein,* dissolve) lyo-.
>
> *Ex*: lyo-enzyme (an enzyme dissolved in the protoplasm of a cell); lyo-philic (dissolving readily); lyo-phobe (a substance which does not dissolve readily); lyo-tropic (easily dissolved).

soul. See under *mind.*

sound (voice sound).

> (Gr. *phone,* sound) phon-; -phone; phono-; -phony.
>
> *Ex*: phon-asthenia (feebleness of the voice); osteo-phone (a type of hearing aid); phono-phobia (fear of loud sounds); broncho-phony (a kind of sound produced in the chest).

sour. See under *acid.*

spasm.

(Gr. *spasma,* a spasm; genit. *spasmatos*) -spasm-; spasmato-; spasmo-.

Ex: arterio-spasm (a spasm of an artery); pyloro-spasm (spasm of the pylorus); spasmato-logy (the study of spasms); spasmogenic (causing spasm); spasmo-lysis (the relief or checking of a spasm).

speech (speech organs; babble).

(Gr. *lalein,* speak) lal-; lali-; lalo-.

Ex: lal-iatry (treatment of speech defects); lalo-phobia (fear of speaking); lalo-plegia (paralysis of the organs of speech).

speech (utterance).

(Gr. *phasis,* speech) -phasia.

Ex: dys-phasia (impairment of speech); brady-phasia (abnormal slowness of speech); a-phasia (loss of the power of speech, etc.). See also *word.*

sperm. See under *semen* and *spermatozoa.*

spermatozoa (sperm; seed).

(Gr. *sperma,* seed; genit; *spermatos*) -sperm-; spermat-; spermato-; spermo-; spermi-.

Ex: sperm-agglutination (agglutination of spermatozoa); spermat-itis (inflammation of a vas deferens); spermato-cyte (an early cell from which a spermatozoon develops); spermato-logy (the study of spermatozoa); spermo-lytic (causing dissolution of spermatozoa); spermi-cidal (causing destruction of spermatozoa).

sphenoid bone (wedge; wedge-shaped).

(Gr. *sphen,* wedge) spheno-; sphen-.

Ex: spheno-cephaly (a condition in which the head has a wedge-shaped appearance); sphen-oid (wedge-shaped); sphenomaxillary (pertaining to the sphenoid bone and the maxilla); sphen-osis (a condition in which the fetus is wedged in the pelvis).

spherical. See under *round.*

sphincter.

(Gr. *sphinkter,* that which draws close) sphincter-; sphinctero-.

Ex: sphincter-ectomy (excision of a sphincter); sphincter-ismus

(a spasm of a sphincter); sphinctero-plasty (a plastic operation on a sphincter); sphinctero-tomy (a surgical cutting of a
sphincter).

spider (slenderness; spider's web).

(Gr. *arachne,* spider) arachn-; arachno-.

Ex: arachn-idism (poisoning by bite of a spider); arachn-itis
(inflammation of the arachnoid membrane); arachno-dactyly
(long and slender fingers); arachno-phobia.

spinal column. See under *spine* and *vertebra.*

spinal cord.

(L. *medulla,* marrow) medull-; medulli-; medullo-.

Ex: medulli-spinal (pertaining to the spinal cord); medullo-
therapy (prevention of rabies by treatment with the spinal cords
of inoculated rabbits).

spinal cord (medulla spinalis).

(Gr. *myelos,* marrow) myel-; myelo-.

Ex: myel-algia (pain in the spinal cord); myel-atrophy (atrophy
of the spinal cord); myelo-cele (a hernia in which the spinal
cord forms the protruding mass); myelo-encephalitis (inflammation of the spinal cord and the brain). See also *spine.*

spinal nerve root. See under *root.*

spine (spinal column; spinal cord).

(L. *spina,* backbone) -spin-; spini-; spino-.

Ex: spin-algia (pain in the spine); spini-fugal (conveying impulses away from the spinal cord); spini-petal (conveying impulses toward the spinal cord); spino-bulbar (pertaining to the
spinal cord and the medulla oblongata).

spine (spinal column; vertabral column).

(Gr. *rachis,* spine) rachi-; rachio-.

Ex: rachi-algia (pain in the spine); rachio-campsis (curvature
of the spine); rachio-pathy (any disease of the spinal column);
rachi-tomy (a surgical cutting into the spinal column).

spirilla.

(L. *spirillum,* small coil) spirill-; spirilli-; spirillo-.

Ex: spirill-emia (presence of spirilla in the blood); spirilli-cide
(a substance which kills spirilla); spirillo-lysis (lysis or destruction of spirilla).

spirochete.

(Gr. *speira*, soil; *chaite*, hair) spirochet-; spirocheti-; spirocheto-. *Ex*: spirochet-emia (presence of spirochetes in the blood); spirocheti-cide (a substance which kills spirochetes); spirocheto-lysis (lysis or destruction of spirochetes).

spleen.

(Gr. *splen*, spleen) splen-; spleni-; spleno-. *Ex*: splen-algia (pain in the spleen); spleni-form (shaped like a spleen); splen-itis (inflammation of the spleen); spleno-ptosis (a downward displacement of the spleen).

spleen (lien).

(L. *lien*, spleen) lien-; lieno-. *Ex*: lien-itis (inflammation of the spleen); lien-ectomy (excision of the spleen); lieno-renal (pertaining to the spleen and the kidney).

split. See under *cleft*.

sponge (sponge-like tissue).

(Gr. *spongia*, sponge) spongi-; spongio-. *Ex*: spongi-form (resembling a sponge); spongi-itis (inflammation of the corpus spongiosum); spongio-blast; spongio-plasm (the network of fibrils forming the reticulum of certain cells).

spore (reproductive cell).

(Gr. *spora*, seed) -spore; spor-; sporo-; spori-. *Ex*: macro-spore (a large spore); spor-angium (a cyst or capsule containing spores); spori-cide (a substance which destroys spores); sporo-genic (producing spores); sporo-mycosis (infection with the spores of a fungus).

sprout (bud; primordium).

(L. *germen*, offshoot) germin-; germino-; germo-. *Ex*: germin-al (in an embryonic stage); germin-ation (a sprouting or beginning of growth); germo-gen (protoplasm from which a reproductive cell arises).

spur. See under *excite*.

spurious. See under *false*.

squama (plate-like structure; scale).

(L. *squama*, a scale) squam-; squamat-; squamo-. *Ex*: squam-ate (resembling a scale or squama); squamatization (a change to a squamous type); squamo-temporal (pertaining to the squamous portion of the temporal bone); de-squam-ation (shedding of the skin in scales).

stalk. See under *peduncle*.

standing (arresting).

(Gr. *stasis,* standing) stasi-; -stasis; -static.

Ex: stasi-phobia (fear of standing); hemo-stasis (arrest of a flow of blood); bacterio-stasis (arrest of the growth of bacteria); ortho-static (standing upright).

stapes

(L. *stapes,* stirrup; genit. *stapedis*) staped-; stapedi-; stapedio-.

Ex: staped-ectomy (excision of the stapes); stapedio-plasty (a plastic operation on the stapes); stapedio-vestibular (pertaining to the stapes and the vestibule).

staphylococcus

(Gr. *staphyle,* bunch of grapes; *kokkos,* berry) staphylococc-; staphylo-.

Ex: staphylococc-al (pertaining to staphylococci); staphylococc-emia (the presence of staphylococci in the blood); staphylo-dermatitis (inflammation of the skin caused by staphylococci); staphylo-lysin (a lysin produced by staphylococci).

starch.

(Gr. *amylon,* starch) amyl-; amylo-.

Ex: amyl-ase (an emzyme which aids in the splitting of starch); amylo-lytic (causing the lysis of starch); amylo-psin (an enzyme which converts starch into maltose).

starvation. See under *hunger*.

stealing (theft).

(Gr. *kleptein,* to steal) klept-; klepti-; kleptio-.

Ex: klepto-lagnia (sexual pleasure derived from stealing); klepto-mania (a compulsion to steal); klept-amnesia (a defense mechanism by which an act of stealing is forgotten).

stem. See under *peduncle*.

stench (rank odor; malodorous).

(Gr. *bromos,* stench) brom-; bromo-.

Ex: brom-hidrosis (malodorous perspiration); bromo-menorrhea (offensive menstrual discharge); bromo-pnea (unpleasant breath).

step. See under *walk.*

sternum (breastbone).

(Gr. *sternon,* sternum) stern-; sterno-.

Ex: stern-ad (toward the sternum); retro-stern-al (behind the sternum); sterno-costal (pertaining to the sternum and the ribs); sterno-clavicular (pertaining to the sternum and the clavicle).

stimulating (exciting; provoking).

(Gr. *erethizein,* arouse) ereth-; erethi-; erethis-; erethiso-.

Ex: ereth-ism (excessive excitability); erethiso-phrenia (excessive mental excitability); erethiso-gastria (excitability of the stomach).

stimulating. See under *inducing* and *turning.*

stomach (abdomen).

(Gr. *gaster,* stomach) gastr-; gastri-; gastro-.

Ex: gastr-algia (pain in the stomach); gastr-ectomy (excision of the stomach); gastro-enteritis (inflammation of the stomach and the intestine); gastro-scopy (inspection of the stomach).

stone (calculus; concretion).

(Gr. *lithos,* stone) lith-; litho-.

Ex: lith-iasis (the presence or formation of calculi); litho-tomy (a surgical incision for the removal of a stone); litho-trite (an instrument for crushing a calculus).

stony. See under *hard.*

stool. See under *feces.*

stoppage (suppression; checking; deficiency).

(Gr. *ischein,* suppress) isch-; ischo-.

Ex: ischo-cholia (suppression of the secretion of bile); ischo-galactic (suppressing the formation of milk in the breast); ischo-menia (stoppage of the menses); isch-emia (a deficiency of blood in a structure).

straight (erected).

(Gr. *ithys,* straight) ithy-; ithyo-.

Ex: ithy-lordosis (lordosis not associated with a lateral curva-

ture); ithy-phallic (pertaining to the erected phallus); ithyo-
kyphosis (kyphosis not associated with a lateral curvature).

straight. See under *normal.*

strange. See under *new.*

strange. See under *foreign.*

strength.

(Gr. *sthenos,* strength) -sthen-; stheno-.

Ex: a-sthen-ia (lack of strength); hypo-sthen-ia (decreased
strength of the body); stheno-meter (an instrument to measure
muscular strength); stheno-phoria (a feeling of strength).

strength. See under *power.*

streptococcus.

(Gr. *streptos,* twisted; *kokkos,* berry) streptococc-; streptococci-;
streptococco-; strepto-.

Ex: streptococc-al (pertaining to streptococci); streptococci-cide
(an agent destructive to streptococci); streptococco-lysin (a
hemolysin produced by streptococci); strepto-derma (a skin infection caused by streptococci).

striated muscle fiber (rod-like structure).

(Gr. *rhabdos,* a rod) rhabd-; rhabdo-.

Ex: rhabd-oid (shaped like a rod); rhabdo-myoma (a tumor
derived from striated muscle fibers); rhabdo-pod (a clasper of
an insect).

stricture (narrowing).

(L. *stringere,* draw tight; pp. *strictus*) strictur-; stricturo-.
Ex: stricturo-genic (inducing the formation of strictures);
stricturo-scope (an instrument designed for the examination of
strictures); stricturo-tome (a surgical knife designed to cut
strictures).

string. See under *cord.*

striving. See under *appetite.*

stroke. See under *paralysis.*

study of. See under *science of.*

stupor (sleep; lethargy; numbness; torpor; insensibility).

(Gr. *narke,* numbness) narco-.

Ex: narco-analysis (psychoanalysis applied to a patient who
is under the effect of a narcotic); narco-lepsy (an uncontrollable

desire to sleep); narco-mania (a mania for narcotics); narco-synthesis (a form of psychiatric treatment in which the patient is under the influence of a barbiturate).

styloid process.

(L. *stilus,* a stake) stylo-.

Ex: stylo-hyoid (pertaining to the styloid process and the hyoid); stylo-mandibular (pertaining to the styloid process and the mandible); stylo-mastoid (pertaining to the styloid process and the mastoid process).

substance. See under *matter.*

suet. See under *fat.*

sugar (carbohydrate; glycogen).

(Gr. *glykys,* sweet) glyc-; glyco-; glycogen-.

Ex: hypo-glyc-emia (decrease in blood sugar); glyco-lytic (breaking down sugars); glyco-neo-genesis (formation of new sugar, from non-sugar material); glycogen-ic (pertaining to glycogen).

sugar (saccharum).

(Gr. *sakcharon,* sugar) -sacchar-; sacchari-; saccharo-.

Ex: sacchar-ide (a carbohydrate); mono-sacchar-ide (a simple sugar); sacchari-meter (a device for determining the amount of sugar in a solution); saccharo-lytic (capable of decomposing sugar); saccharo-lysis (decomposition of sugar).

sulfur.

(Gr. *theion,* sulfur) thio-.

Ex: Thio-bacterium (a genus of microorganisms capable of oxidizing sulfur compounds); thio-glucose (a sugar containing sulfur); thio-philic (thriving in the presence of sulfur).

sun (sunlight).

(Gr. *helios,* sun) heli-; helio-.

Ex: heli-ation (treatment by exposure to sunlight); helio-phobia (fear of, or sensitivity to, sunlight); helio-tropism (tropism caused by sunlight).

sun (sunlight).

(L. *sol,* sun; *solaris,* pertaining to the sun) sol-; solar-; solo-.

Ex: solar-ize (to submit to the action of sunlight); solo-genous (caused by the sun); sol-arium (a room suitable for exposing the body to the sun).

suppression. See under *stoppage.*

surrounding. See under *around.*

suturing (sewing together).

(Gr. *rhaphe,* a seam) -rrhaphy.

Ex: teno-rrhaphy (surgical suturing of a cut tendon); neuro-rrhaphy (the suturing of a cut or torn nerve); myo-rrhaphy (the suturing of a cut muscle); episio-rrhaphy (the suturing of a lacerated perineum).

swallowing (deglutition).

(L. *deglutire,* swallow) deglutit-; deglutiti-; -gluti.

Ex: deglutit-ion (swallowing); deglutit-ory (pertaining to swallowing); dys-gluti-a (difficult swallowing); deglutit-odynia (painful swallowing).

sweat (perspiration).

(Gr. *hidros,* sweat) -hidr-; hidro-; hidrot-.

Ex: hidr-adenitis (inflammation of sweat glands); hidro-poiesis (production of sweat); caco-hidr-osis (any disorder in sweat production); hyper-hidr-osis (excessive perspiration); an-hidrot-ic (a substance which checks perspiration).

sweat (perspiration).

(L. *sudor,* sweat) sudor-; sudori-; sudoro-.

Ex: sudor-al (pertaining to sweat); sudor-esis (profuse perspiration); sudori-ferous (conveying perspiration); sudoro-genous (caused by sweat).

swelling (tumor).

(Gr. *oidema,* swelling) edem-; edema-; edemat-; edemati-; edemato-.

Ex: edemati-zation (the process of becoming swollen); edemat-ous; edemato-genic (producing edema). See also *tumor.*

swift. See under *rapid.*

swing. See under *oscillate.*

sympathetic nervous system (sympathetic nerve).

(Gr. *sympathetikos,* sympathetic) sympath-; sympatheo-; sympathet-; sympathetic-; sympathetico-.

Ex: sympath-ectomy (resection of a sympathetic nerve);

sympatheo-neuritis (neuritis involving a sympathetic nerve); sympathet-ic; sympathetic-algia (pain in a sympathetic nerve or ganglion); sympathetico-tonia (excessive activity or dominance of the sympathetic nervous system).

synovial membrane (synovia).

(Gr. *syn*, with; L. *ovum*, egg) synov-; synovi-; synovio-.

Ex: synov-ectomy (surgical excision of a synovial membrane); synovi-al; synovi-analysis (analysis of synovial fluid); synovio-blast (a fibrous cell or fibroblast of a synovial membrane).

syphilis.

(Gr. *siphlos*, crippled) syphil-; syphilo-.

Ex: syphil-id (cutaneous eruption due to syphilis); syphilo-genous (caused by syphilis); syphilo-graphy (a treatise on syphilis); syphilo-therapy (treatment of syphilis).

systole.

(Gr. *systole*, contraction) systol-; -systole; systolo-.

Ex: a-systole (incomplete or absent contraction of the ventricles); holo-systol-ic (pertaining to the entire systole); tele-systol-ic (pertaining to the last part of a systole); pre-systol-ic (occurring before a systole).

T

tail (tail-like appendage).

(L. *cauda*, tail) caud-; cauda-; caudo-.

Ex: caud-ad (toward the tail); caudo-cephalad (from the tail toward the head).

tallow. See under *fat.*

talus (ankle bone).

(L. *talus*, ankle) talo-.

Ex: talo-calcaneal (pertaining to the talus and the calcaneus); talo-fibular (pertaining to the talus and the fibula); talo-navicular (pertaining to the talus and the navicular).

tapeworm.

(L. *taenia*, tapeworm) teni-; tenia-; tenio-.

Ex: teni-form (resembling a tapeworm); tenia-cide (an agent destructive to tapeworms); tenio-toxin (a toxin produced by tapeworms).

tapping. See under *perforation.*

tarsus of ankle.

(Gr. *tarsos,* flat surface) -tars-; tarso-; -tarsus.

Ex: tars-algia (pain in the ankle); tarso-phalangeal (pertaining to the tarsus and toes or phalanges); tarso-tibial (pertaining to the tarsus and the tibia).

tarsus of eyelid.

(Gr. *tarsos,* flat surface) -tars-; tarso-.

Ex: tars-itis (inflammation of the tarsus of the eyelid); tarso-malacia (abnormal softening of the tarsus of the eyelid); tarso-plasty (a plastic operation on the tarsus of an eyelid).

taste (sense of taste).

(L. *gustare,* to taste; Gr. *geusis,* taste) gust-; gustat-; geus-; -geusia.

Ex: gust-ation (act of tasting); gustat-ory (pertaining to the sense of taste); oxy-geusia (sharpness of the sense of taste); hypo-geusia (dullness of the sense of taste); a-geusia (loss of the sense of taste).

tears (lacrimal apparatus).

(Gr. *dakryon,* a tear) dacry-; dacryo-.

Ex: dacry-ops (a watery or teary condition of the eye); dacryo-rrhea (copious flow of tears); dacryo-cyst (lacrimal sac).

tears (tear fluid).

(L. *lacrima,* tear) lacrim-; lacrima-; lacrimo-.

Ex: lacrim-al (pertaining to tears); lacrim-ation (discharge of tears); lacrimo-nasal (pertaining to the lacrimal apparatus and the nose).

temple. See under *temporal bone.*

temporal bone (temple).

(L. *tempus,* temple; pl. *tempora*) tempor-; temporo-.

Ex: tempor-al (pertaining to the temple); temporo-mandibular (pertaining to the temporal bone and the mandible); temporo-parietal (pertaining to the temporal and parietal bones).

ten (tenfold).

(Gr. *deka,* ten) deca-.

Ex: deca-meter (ten meters); deca-curie (ten curies); deca-liter.

tendon.

(L. *tendo,* tendon; Gr. *tenon,* tendon) tendin-; tendino-; tendo-; teno-; tenon-; tenonto-.

Ex: tendin-itis (inflammation of a tendon); tendino-plasty (a plastic operation on a tendon); tendo-lysis (the surgical freeing of a tendon from adhesions); tendo-vaginal (pertaining to a tendon and tendon sheath); teno-myotomy (excision of a part of a tendon and a muscle); tenon-ectomy (excision of a part of a tendon); tenonto-graphy (a description of tendons).

tension.

(L. *tensio,* tension) tensio-; -tension.

Ex: tensio-meter (an instrument for measuring tension); tensio-genous (caused by tension); hyper-tension; hypo-tension; normo-tension (normal tension). See also *tone.*

tenth. See under *one-tenth.*

term. See under *name.*

termination. See under *end.*

testicle (testis).

(Gr. *orchis,* testis) orch-; orchi-; orchid-; orchido-; orchio-.

Ex: orchi-algia (pain in a testicle); orchid-ectomy (surgical removal of a testicle); orchido-tomy (a surgical cutting into a testicle); orchio-plasty (a plastic operation on a testicle). See also *testis*

testis (testicle).

(L. *testis,* male gonad; *testiculus,* male gonad) test-; testi-; testicul-; testo-.

Ex: test-algia (pain in a testicle); testi-cond (having the testicles within the abodmen); testicul-oma (a tumor of the testicle); testo-pathy (any disease of a testicle).

tetanus.

(Gr. *tetanos,* spasm) tetan-; tetani-; tetano-.

Ex: tetan-ic (pertaining to tetanus); tetani-form (resembling tetanus); tetani-genic (producing tetanus); tetano-toxin (the toxin of tetanus).

thalamus.

(Gr. *thalamos,* inner chamber) thalam-; thalamo-.

Ex: thalam-ic (pertaining to the thalamus); thalamo-cortical

(pertaining to the thalamus and the cortex); thalamo-tegmental
(pertaining to the thalamus and the tegmentum).

theft. See under *stealing.*

therapy (treatment).

(Gr. *therapeuein,* take care of) therap-; therapeut-; -therapy.
Ex: therap-ist (a person trained in the treatment of disease);
therapeut-ics (the science of treating disease); balneo-therapy
(the use of baths in the treatment of disease); hydro-therapy
(the use of water in the treatment of disease).

thick (compact; solid; frequent).

(Gr. *pyknos,* thick) pykn-; pykno-.
Ex: pykn-ic (having a thick, stocky build); pykno-morphous
(having compact stainable elements); pykn-osis (a shrinking
and thickening of a nucleus).

thick (thickened; dense).

(Gr. *pachys,* thick) pachy-.
Ex: pachy-blepharon (a thickening of an eyelid); pachy-derma
(a thickening of the skin); pachy-meninx (the dura mater);
pachy-vaginitis (inflammation of the vagina associated with a
thickening of the tissues).

thin. See under *slender.*

third.

(L. *tertius,* third) terti-.
Ex: terti-an (recurring every third day); terti-gravida (a woman who has had three childbirths in three pregnancies).

thorax. See under *chest.*

thousand (thousand times).

(Gr. *chilioi,* thousand) kilo-.
Ex: kilo-calorie (large calorie; a thousand calories); kilo-cycle
(a thousand cycles per second); kilo-gram (a thousand grams).

thousandth. See under *one thousandth.*

thread (thread-like).

(Gr. *mitos,* thread) mit-; mito-.
Ex: mito-chondria (rod-shaped structures occurring in cyto-
plasm); mit-osis (a form of cell division in which the chromatin
forms a thread-like structure); mito-genic (causing mitosis).

thread (threadworm).

(L. *filum,* thread) fil-; filar-; filari-.

Ex: fil-ar (resembling a thread); filari-al (pertaining to thread-worms); filar-iasis (infestation with threadworms or filariae).

thread. See under *nematode.*

threadworm. See under *pinworm* and *thread.*

three (three times).

(Gr. *treis,* three) tri-.

Ex: tri-acetate (a compound containing three acetic acid groups); tri-atomic (composed of three atoms); tri-laminar (composed of three layers).

three-dimensional. See under *solid.*

throat. See under *neck* and *pharynx.*

thrombus.

(Gr. *thrombos,* thrombus) thromb-; thrombo-.

Ex: thromb-ectomy (excision of a thrombus); thrombo-genesis (the formation of thrombi); thrombo-lytic (tending to dissolve thrombi); thrombo-philia (a predisposition to the development of thrombi).

through (across; apart; between).

(Gr. *dia,* through) di-; dia-.

Ex: dia-dermic (through the skin); dia-lysis (separation by passage through a membrane); dia-pedesis (passage of cells through the wall of a blood vessel); di-uresis (passage of urine through the kidneys; excessive urination).

through (throughout; completely; excessively).

(L. *per,* through) per-.

Ex: per-acute (marked by excessive acuteness); per-colate (to allow a solvent to trickle through a medicinal substance); per-cutaneous (through the skin). See also *across.*

throughout. See under *through.*

thumb.

(L. *pollex,* thumb; genit. *pollicis*) pollic-; pollici-.

Ex: pollic-ectomy (the surgical removal of the thumb); pollic-ization (the reconstruction of the index finger into a thumb); pollici-form (having the shape of a thumb).

thymus gland.

> (Gr. *thymos,* thymus) thymo-.
> *Ex*: thymo-cyte (a cell occurring in the thymus); thymo-kinetic (stimulating the thymus); thymo-privous (caused by removal of the thymus).

thyroid gland.

> (Gr. *thyreos,* shield) thyro-; thyroid-.
> *Ex*: thyro-aplasia (incomplete development of the thyroid); thyro-genous (caused by the thyroid); thyroid-itis (inflammation of the thyroid gland); hyper-thyroid-ism; thyro-toxin (a toxin produced by the thyroid).

tibia.

> (L. *tibia,* shinbone) tibi-; tibio-.
> *Ex*: tibi-algia (pain in the tibia); tibio-fibular (pertaining to the tibia and the fibula); tibio-navicular (pertaining to the tibia and the navicular bone).

time (duration).

> (Gr. *chronos,* time) chron-; chroni; chrono-.
> *Ex*: chron-icity (the condition of being chronic); chrono-graph (instrument for recording intervals of time); chrono-tropic (affecting the duration or rate); syn-chron-ous (happening simultaneously).

tint. See under *color.*

tip. See under *limb.*

tissue (web).

> (Gr. *histos,* web) hist-; histi-; histio-; histo-.
> *Ex*: hist-affine (having an affinity for tissues); histio-cyte (a cell of the reticuloendothelial system); histo-logy (the study of tissues); histo-lysis (the lysis of tissues).

to (toward; near; together).

> (L. *ad,* to) ac- (before letter *c* or *q*); af- (before *f*); ag- (before *g*); al- (before *l*); an- (before *n*); ap- before *p*); ar- (before *r*); as- before *s*); at- (before *t*); ad- (before most other letters).
> *Ex*: ac-cessory (supplementary to another); ad-nerval (toward a nerve); ad-sternal (toward the sternum); af-ferent (conveying toward or to); ag-glomerate (to mass together); al-ligation (a

method of mixing medicinal solutions); an-nectent (joining together); ap-pendage (something added to); ar-rector (muscle which raises up to); as-similation (transformation to living matter); at-traction (a drawing toward).

toe. See under *digit.*

toe, great.

(L. *hallux,* great toe; genit. *hallucis*) halluc-; halluci-; halluco-. *Ex*: halluc-al (pertaining to the great toe); halluci-form (resembling the great toe); halluco-plasty (a plastic operation on the great toe).

toenail. See under *nail.*

together. See under *with.*

toil. See under *work.*

tone (tonus; tension).

(Gr. *tonos,* tension) -ton-; tono-.

Ex: hyper-ton-ic (having high tension); a-ton-y (lack of tone); tono-clonic (tonic and clonic); tono-meter (an instrument to measure tension); tono-genous (caused by tension).

tongue (lingua).

(L. *lingua,* tongue) lingu-; lingui-. *Ex*: sub-lingu-al (under the tongue); e-lingu-ation (excision of the tongue); lingui-form (shaped like a tongue).

tongue (tongue-shaped structure).

(Gr. *glossa,* tongue; Attic Gr. *glotta,* tongue) gloss-; glosso-; glott-; glotto-. *Ex*: gloss-algia (pain in the tongue); gloss-itis (inflammation of the tongue); glosso-plegia (paralysis of the tongue); glotto-logy (study of the tongue); macro-gloss-ia (enlargement of the tongue).

tonsil.

(L. *tonsilla,* tonsil) tonsill-; tonsillo-. *Ex*: tonsill-ar (pertaining to a tonsil); tonsill-ectomy; tonsillo-lith (a concretion formed in a tonsil); tonsillo-pathy (any disease of a tonsil).

tonus. See under *tone.*

tooth (dens).

(Gr. *odon.* tooth; genit. *odontos*) odont-; odontin-; odonto-; -odontia; -odontics; -odontist.

Ex: odont-ectomy (excision of a tooth); odontin-oid (resembling a tooth or tooth substance); odonto-scope (a small mirror used by dentists for inspecing the teeth); orth-odontia (dentistry dealing with irregularities of teeth); orth-odontics; orth-odontist (a practitioner of orthodontia).

tooth (involving teeth).

(L. *dens,* tooth; genit. *dentis*) dent-; denta-; denti-; dento-; **-dentia.**

Ex: dent-algia (pain in a tooth or teeth); denti-lingual (pertaining to the teeth and tongue); denti-tion (arrangement of the teeth; eruption of the teeth); dento-legal (pertaining to dentistry and the law); e-dentia (toothlessness).

torpor. See under *stupor.*

tortuous. See under *varix.*

touch (feel with the hand; palpate).

(L. *palpare,* touch) palp-; palpa-; palpato-.

Ex: palp-able (perceptible to the touch); palp-ation; palpato-metry (measurement of pressure caused by touch); palpato-genous (caused by touching or palpating).

touch (sense of touch).

(L. *tangere,* to touch; pp. *tactus*) -tact-; tacto-; tactil-.

Ex: tact-ile (pertaining to the sense of touch); a-tactil-ia (loss of the sense of touch); tacto-meter (an instrument used to measure the sharpness of the sense of touch).

touch (seizure; contact).

(Gr. *haptein,* to touch) hapt-; hapto-.

Ex: hapt-ics (the study of the sense of touch); hapto-meter (an instrument used to test the sensitivity to touch); hapto-phobia (fear of being touched).

touch (touch perception).

(Gr. *haphe,* touch) haphe-; -aph-.

Ex: haph-algesia (sensation of pain caused by being touched or by touching); haphe-phobia (abnormal fear of being touched); hypo-aph-ia (decreased sensitivity to touch); dys-aph-ia (impairment of the sense of touch); oxy-aph-ia (sharpness of the sense of touch).

touch sensation.

(Gr. *thigma,* touch) thigm-; thigmo-.

Ex: hypo-thigm-ia (a diminished sensitivity to touch); hyper-thigm-ia; thigm-esthesia (the perception of the stimulus of touch); thigmo-taxis (movement of an organism or part in response to touch).

toward (against; over; in front).

(L. *ob,* against) ob-; o- (before *m*); oc- (before *c*); of- (before *f*); op- (before *p*).

Ex: ob-literate (to remove completely); oc-clude (to bring together); op-pilative (tending to obstruct or constipate).

toward (in direction of).

(L. *ad,* to) -ad.

Ex: cephal-ad (toward the head); dors-ad (toward the dorsum); ventr-ad (toward the front); caud-ad (toward the tail or lower end); proxim-ad (toward the near end).

toward. See under *to.*

toxin (poison).

(Gr. *toxikon;* L. *toxinum*) -tox-; toxi-; toxico-; toxo-; toxin-; toxini-.

Ex: tox-albumin (a toxic albumin); tox-emia; toxico-dendrol (a poisonous oil); toxico-logy (the study of poisons and toxins); toxini-cide (a substance which destroys a toxin); toxo-protein (a toxic protein).

trachea.

(Gr. *tracheia arteria,* rough windpipe) trache-; trachea-; tracheo-.

Ex: trache-algia (pain in the trachea); tracheo-cele (herniation of a portion of the tracheal mucosa); tracheo-genic originating in the trachea); tracheo-malacia (softening of the trachea); tracheo-tomy.

tracing (recording; letter; writing).

(Gr. *gramma,* something written) -gram.

Ex: encephalo-gram (an x-ray picture of the brain or head); electrocardio-gram; sphygmo-gram (a tracing of the pulse);

roentgeno-gram (an x-ray picture); pelmato-gram (a footprint); dactylo-gram (a fingerprint).

transformation. See under *mutation.*

translucent. See under *glass.*

transposed. See under *changed.*

trauma (injury).

(G. *trauma,* injury) trauma-; traumato-; traumat-.

Ex: trauma-therapy (treatment of injuries); traumat-ism (the general disorder resulting from an injury); traumato-genic (causing trauma); traumato-logy (the study of injuries).

treatment. See under *physician* and *therapy.*

treponema.

(Gr. *trepein,* to turn; *nema,* thread) treponem-; treponemat-; treponemi-.

Ex: treponem-iasis (infection of the body with treponemas); treponemat-osis (the abnormal condition resulting from infection with treponemas); treponemi-cidal (destructive to treponemas).

tribe (clan; phylum).

(Gr. *phylon,* race) -phyl-; phylo-.

Ex: phylo-geny (the history of the development of a race); phylo-logy (The study of races); phylo-graphy (a treatise describing races); neo-phylic (pertaining to a new race); poly-phyl-etic (derived from several kinds of races).

trichina. See under *trichinella.*

trichinella (trichina).

(Gr. *trichinos,* hairy) trichinell-; trichini-; trichino-.

Ex: trichinell-iasis (infestation with trichinae); trichini-ferous (bearing trichinae); trichino-phobia (abnormal fear of infestation with trichinae).

trochanter.

(Gr. *trochanter,* trochanter) -trochanter-; trochantero-.

Ex: intra-trochanter-ic (between the trochanters); infra-trochanteric; trochanter-ectomy (excision of a trochanter); trochantero-plasty (a plastic operation on a trochanter).

trochlea (pulley).

(Gr. *trochilia,* sheaf of a pulley) trochleari-; -trochle-; trochleo-.
Ex: trochleari-form (shaped like a trochlea or pulley); supra-trochle-ar (situated above the trochlea); trochleo-plasty (a plastic operation on a trochlea).

trypanosome.

(Gr. *trypanon,* borer; *soma,* body) trypan-; trypano-; trypanosom-; trypanosomat-; tryponosomato-; tryanosomi-;
Ex: trypan-id (the eruption occurring in trypanosomiasis); trypano-lytic (destructive to trypanosomes); trypanosom-iasis (infection with trypanosomes); trypanosomat-ic (pertaining to trypanosomes); trypanosomato-tropic (having an affinity for trypanosomes); trypanosomi-cide (a substance destructive to trypanosomes).

trypsin.

(Gr. *tripsis,* a rubbing; *pepsin*) trypsin-; trypsino; trypt-; trypto-.
Ex: trypsin-ize (to treat with trypsin); trypsino-gen (the precursor of trypsin); trypt-ic (pertaining to the action of trypsin); trypto-lytic (pertaining to the splitting function of trypsin).

tube (auditory tube; uterine tube).

(Gr. *salpinx,* trumpet; genit. *salpingos*) salping-; salpingo-.
Ex: salping-ectomy (excision of a uterine tube); salping-itis (inflammation of a uterine tube or an auditory tube); salpingo-oophoritis (inflammation of a uterine tube and an ovary).

tube (fistula).

(Gr. *syrinx,* tube; genit. *syringos*) syring-; syringo-.
Ex: syring-ectomy (the excision of a fistula); syringo-bulbia (formation of cavities in the medulla oblongata); syringo-myelia (cavitation of the spinal cord).

tube (uterine tube; auditory tube).

(L. *tubus,* a pipe) tubo-.
Ex: tubo-abdominal (pertaining to the uterine tubes and the abdomen); tubo-ovarian (pertaining to a uterine tube and an ovary); tubo-rrhea (a profuse discharge from an auditory tube).

tubercle.

(L. *tuberculum,* small knob or nodule) tubercul-.

Ex: tubercul-ar (pertaining to tubercles); tubercul-ated (covered with tubercles); tubercul-ectomy (excision of a tubercle).

tuberculin.

(L. *tuberculum,* small knob or nodule; *-in*) tuberculin-; tuberculino-.

Ex: tuberculin-ization (the application of tuberculin); tuberculino-therapy (the use of tuberculin in therapy); tuberculino-genous (caused by the action of tuberculin).

tuberculosis.

(L. *tuberculum,* small knob; *-osis,* abnormal condition) tubercul-; tuberculo-.

Ex: tubercul-id (a skin lesion occurring in tuberculosis); tuberculo-static (slowing or checking the progress of tuberculosis); tuberculo-tropic (having an affinity for the tubercle bacillus); tuberculo-derm (tuberculous disease of the skin).

tuberculosis. See under *wasting.*

tuft. See under *crest* and *villus.*

tumor (neoplasm; mass; growth).

(Gr. *onkoma,* swelling) -oma; *pl.* -omata.

Ex: hemat-oma (a mass or tumor containing blood); ele-oma (tumor caused by an injection of oil into a tissue); syphil-oma (a tumor caused by syphilis); hemangi-oma (a tumor composed of blood vessels); myel-oma (a tumor of bone marrow).

tumor (neoplasm; mass; swelling).

(Gr. *onkos,* mass) onco-.

Ex: onco-genesis (the development of tumors); onco-logy (the study of tumors); onco-tomy (the cutting of a swelling or tumor).

turn (change).

(L. *vertere,* turn; pp. *versus*) -vers-; versi-; -version.

Ex: versi-color (changing color); re-vers-al; retro-version (the turning of the uterus backward); antero-version (a turning of the uterus forward).

turning (changing; stimulating).

(Gr. *trope,* a turning) -trop-; trope; -tropic; -tropia; -tropism; tropo-.

Ex: trop-agnosia (inability to perceive change in position); gonado-trope (a substance which stimulates the gonads); adreno-tropic (stimulating the adrenal glands); eso-tropia (a turning of the eyeball inward); helio-tropism (a turning or changing in response to light); tropo-philous (thriving under changing conditions). See also *rotation.*

twin (twins; twinning).

(L. *geminus,* twin; *gemellus,* diminutive of *geminus*) gemin-; gemini-; gemino-; gemell-; gemelli-; gemello-.

Ex: bi-gemin-al (paired); gemelli-para (a woman who has borne twins); gemello-logy (study of twinning).

twisted (twisted chain; curved).

(Gr. *streptos,* twisted) strept-; strepto-.

Ex: strepto-bacteria (bacteria occurring in the form of twisted chains); strepto-cocci (cocci occurring in pairs or chains); Strepto-neura (a group of mollusks having a loop of twisted visceral nerves).

twisted. See under *curved.*

twisting. See under *rotation.*

two (twice; double).

(L. *bi,* two) bi-; bis-.

Ex: bi-cuspid (having two cusps or points); bi-nomial (composed of or designated by two names); bis-axillary (pertaining to both axillae).

two (twice; double).

(Gr. *dis,* twice) di-.

Ex: di-atomic (composed of two atoms); di-basic (containing two hydrogen atoms that can be replaced by bases); di-cephalus (a fetal monster having two heads); di-crotic (having two waves); di-saccharide (double sugar).

twofold. See under *double.*

tympanum (middle ear).

(Gr. *tympanon,* drum) tympan-; tympano-.

Ex: tympan-itis (inflammation of the middle ear); tympano-

mandibular (pertaining to the middle ear and the mandible);
tympano-stapedial (pertaining to the middle ear and the stapes).

typhoid

(Gr. *typhos,* a vapor) typho-; typhoid-.

Ex: typho-bacterin (a type of typhoid vaccine); typho-mania
(a delirium associated with typhoid fever); typho-pneumonia
(typhoid fever and pneumonia); typhoid-al (pertaining to or
resembling typhoid fever).

U

ulcer.

(L. *ulcus,* ulcer) ulcer-; ulcero-.

Ex: ulcer-ation (formation of ulcers or an ulcer); ulcero-genic
(causing the formation of an ulcer or ulcers); ulcero-static
(checking the development of an ulcer); ulcero-therapy (the
treatment of ulcers).

ulcer (ulceration).

(Gr. *helkos,* ulcer) helc-; helco-.

Ex: helc-oid (like an ulcer); helc-osis (the formation of ulcers
or an ulcer); helco-plasty (a plastic operation on an ulcer);
helc-ectomy (the surgical excision of an ulcer).

ultraviolet rays.

(L. *ultra,* beyond; *viola,* a violet) uvio-; uviol-.

Ex: uviol-ize (to subject to ultraviolet rays); uvio-resistant
(resisting the effect of ultraviolet rays); uvio-sensitive (sensitive to the action of ultraviolet rays).

umbilicus (navel).

(L. *umbilicus,* navel) umbil-; umbili-; umbilo-.

Ex: umbil-ectomy (excision of the umbilicus); umbili-form
(resembling a navel); umbilo-plasty (a plastic operation on the
navel).

unchanging. See under *same.*

uncovered. See under *nude.*

under (beneath; below; almost; near).

(L. *sub,* under) sub-.

Ex: sub-acromial (below the acromion); sub-astringent (almost or moderately astringent); sub-coracoid (beneath the cora-

coid process); sub-endothelial (beneath an endothelium); sub-liminal (below the threshold). See also *beneath*.

underneath. See under *below*.

unite. See under *join*.

united. See under *with*.

universal. See under *all*.

unrestricted. See under *all*.

unsuccessful. See under *difficult*.

unwrinkled. See under *smooth*.

up (upward; again; excessive).

(Gr. *ana*, up) ana-.

Ex: ana-bolism (a building up of complex substances); ana-crotism (the presence of a notch on ascending limb of the pulse tracing); ana-phase (a stage in mitosis); ana-phoria (a tendency of a visual axis to move upward).

upon. See under *on*.

upper extremity. See under *arm*.

upper jaw. See under *maxilla*.

uppermost part. See under *head*.

upward. See under *up*.

urea.

(Gr. *ouron*, urine) urea-; ureo-.

Ex: urea-meter (an instrument to estimate urea); ureo-lysis (the decomposition of urea); ureo-telic (having urea as the end product).

ureter.

(Gr. *oureter*, ureter) ureter-; uretero-.

Ex: ureter-algia (pain in a ureter); ureter-ectomy (excision of a ureter); uretero-lysis (the freeing of a ureter from adhesions); uretero-pyelitis (inflammation of a ureter and the pelvis of a kidney).

urethra.

(Gr. *ourethra*, urethra) urethr-; urethro-.

Ex: urethr-emphraxis (a blockage or obstruction of the urethra); urethr-ism (a spasm of the urethra); urethro-scope (an instrument for examining the interior of the urethra); urethro-vesical (pertaining to the urethra and the bladder).

urge. See under *excite.*

uric acid.

(Gr. *ourikos,* pertaining to urine) uricacid-; urico-.
Ex: uricacid-emia (presence of excessive amount of uric acid
in the blood); urico-lysis (the lysis of uric acid); urico-telic
(excreted chiefly as uric acid).

urine.

(Gr. *ouron,* urine) -ur-; -uria; urin-; urini-; uro-; urono-.
Ex: ure-emia (the presence of urinary impurities in the blood);
an-uria; urin-able (that may be excreted in the urine); urini-
ferous (conveying urine); uro-bilin (a brownish pigment);
urono-phile (growing in urine).

usage. See under *law.*

U-shaped. See under *hyoid bone.*

usual. See under *normal.*

uterine tube. See under *tube.*

uterus.

(L. *uterus,* uterus) uter-; utero-.
Ex: uter-algia (pain in the uterus); utero-rectal (pertaining to
the uterus and rectum); utero-vaginal (pertaining to the uterus
and the vagina); utero-vesical (pertaining to the uterus and
the bladder).

uterus (womb).

(Gr. *metra,* uterus) metr-; metra-; metro-.
Ex: metr-algia (pain in the uterus); metr-ectasia (dilatation
of the uterus); metro-pathy (any disease of the uterus);
metro-rrhagia (bleeding from the uterus); endo-metr-itis (inflammation of the lining of the uterus).

uterus (womb; hysteria).

(Gr. *hystera,* uterus) hyster-; hysteri-; hysterico-; hystero-.
Ex: hyster-ectomy (excision of the uterus); hysterico-neuralgic
(pertaining to hysteria and neuralgia); hystero-tomy (a surgical cutting into the uterus).

utterance. See under *speech.*

uvea.

(L. *uva,* grape) uve-; uveo-.

Ex: uve-itic (pertaining to the uvea); uve-itis (inflammation of the uvea); uveo-plasty (a plastic operation on the uvea).

uvula.

(Gr. *staphyle,* bunch of grapes)staphyl-; staphylo-.

Ex: staphyl-ectomy (excision of the uvula); staphyl-edema (swelling of the uvula); staphylo-dialysis (abnormal relaxation of the uvula); staphylo-plasty (a plastic operation on the uvula).

uvula.

(L. *uvula,* small grape) uvul-; uvulo-.

Ex: uvul-ectomy (excision of the uvula); uvul-itis; uvulo-ptosis (a sagging of the uvula); uvulo-tomy (surgical cutting of the uvula).

uvula (uvula-like structure).

(Gr. *kion,* uvula) cion-; ciono-.

Ex: cion-itis (inflammation of the uvula); ciono-ptosis (elongation of the uvula).

V

vaccine.

(L. *vaccinus,* vaccine; *vacca,* a cow) vacci-; vaccin-; vaccini-; vaccino-.

Ex: vacci-genous (producing a vaccine); vaccin-able (that may be vaccinated successfully); vaccini-form (like a vaccine); vaccino-therapy (treatment with vaccines).

vagina.

(L. *vagina,* a sheath) vagin-; vagini-; vagino-.

Ex: vagin-ectomy (excision of the vagina); vagini-colinc (inhabiting the vagina); vagin-ismus (spasm of the vagina); vagin-itis; vagino-perineal (pertaining to the vagina and the perineum); vagino-vesical (pertaining to the vagina and the bladder).

vagina (sheath).

(Gr. *koleos,* sheath) cole-; coleo-.

Ex: cole-itis (inflammation of the vagina); coleo-cystitis (inflammation of the vagina and the bladder).

vagina (vaginal canal).

(Gr. *kysthos,* vagina) kysth-; kystho-.

Ex: kysth-itis (inflammation of the vagina); kysth-odynia (pain in the vagina); kystho-phobia (an aversion for the vagina, on the part of a man).

vagina (womb; hollow; fold).

(Gr. *kolpos,* hollow) colp-; colpi-; colpo-.

Ex: colp-algia (pain in the vagina); colp-ectasia (dilatation of the vagina); colpo-cele (herniation into the vagina); colpo-scope (instrument for examining the vagina).

vagus nerve.

(L. *vago,* to wander) vago-.

Ex: vago-mimetic (resembling the effect of vagal stimulation); vago-tomy (the surgical cutting of a vagus nerve); vago-tonia (excessive activity of the vagi).

valve.

(L. *valva,* leaf of door; *valvula,* small door) valv; valvi-; valvo-; valvu-; valvulo-.

Ex: valv-ate (provided with valves); valvi-form (having the shape of a valve); valvo-tomy (the sugical cutting of a valve); valvul-itis (inflammation of a valve); valvulo-plasty (a plastic operation on a valve or valvula).

varicose. See under *varix.*

varied. See under *irregular.*

varix (varicose; tortuous and dilated).

(L. *varix,* enlarged vein; genit. *varicis*) varic-; varici-; varico-.

Ex: varic-eal (pertaining to a varix); varici-form (having the form of a varix); varic-ose; varico-tomy (incision or excision of a varix).

vegetable. See under *plant.*

vein (veins).

(L. *vena,* vein) ven-; veni-; veno-.

Ex: ven-ectasia (dilatation of a vein); veni-puncture (puncture of a vein with a needle); veno-clysis (the injection of medicinal or nutrient solution into a vein).

vein (venous).

(Gr. *phleps,* vein; genit. *phlebos*) phleb-; phlebo-.

Ex: phleb-itis (inflammation of a vein or veins); phleb-ectomy (excision of a vein); phlebo-graphy (the taking of x-ray pictures of veins); phlebo-stasis (a stasis of the blood in the veins).

venereal disease (libido; coitus).

(Gr. *kypris,* Aphrodite) cyprid-; cyprido-.

Ex: cyprido-logy (study of venereal diseases); cyprido-pathy (venereal disease); cyprido-phobia (abnormal fear of venereal disease); cyprido-mania (intense sexual desire).

ventral. See under *abdomen.*

ventricle (cardiac ventricle; brain ventricle).

(L. *ventriculus,* small belly) ventricul-; ventriculo-.

Ex: ventricul-itis (inflammation of a ventricle); ventriculo-gram (an x-ray picture of a cerebral ventricle); ventriculo-puncture (a surgical puncture of a cerebral ventricle).

vertebra

(L. *vertebra,* vertebra) vertebr-; vertebro-.

Ex: vertebr-al (pertaining to a vertebra); vertebr-ate; vertebr-ectomy (excision of a vertebra); vertebro-costal (pertaining to vertebrae and ribs); vertebro-sternal (pertaining to the vertebrae and the sternum).

vertebra (spinal column).

(Gr. *spondylos,* vertebra) spondyl-; spondylo-.

Ex: spondyl-arthritis (arthritis involving the joints between the vertebrae); spondyl-itis (inflammation of vertebrae); spondylo-desis (surgical fusion of vertebrae); spondylo-pathy (any disease of vertebrae).

vertebral column. See under *spine.*

vertigo.

(L. *vertigo,* vertigo) -vertigin-; vertigini-; vertigino-.

Ex: anti-vertigin-al (tending to check vertigo); vertigini-form (resembling vertigo); vertigino-genic (causing vertigo); vertigino-clinic (inclined to have vertigo).

vesicle (blister).

(L. *vesicula,* small bladder) -vesic-; vesico-; vesicul-; vesiculi-; vesiculo-.

Ex: vesic-ant (a substance which causes the formation of blisters); vesic-ation (formation of blisters); vesico-lytic (resolving blisters); vesicul-ation (eruption of vesicles); vesiculiform (having the shape of a vesicle); vesicul-itis (inflammation of a seminal vesicle); vesiculo-papular (marked by both vesicles and papules).

vesicle. See under *blister.*

vessel (blood vessel).

(Gr. *angeion,* vessel) angi-; angio-.

Ex: angi-ectomy (excision of a portion of a vessel); angi-itis (inflammation of a blood vessel); angio-blast (the early tissue from which blood vessels and cells are formed); angio-pathy (a disease of vessels); angio-spasm (a spasm of a blood vessel).

vessel

(L. *vasculum,* small vessel) vascular-; vasculo-.

Ex: vascular-ity (the condition of having blood vessels); vascular-ization (the development of blood vessels); vasculo-lymphatic (pertaining to blood vessels and lymph vessels).

vessel (blood vessel; ductus deferens).

(L. *vas,* vessel) vas-; vasi-; vaso-.

Ex: vas-ectomy (excision of the ductus deferens); vasi-form (resembling a vessel); vaso-construction (constriction of blood vessels); vaso-motor (controlling the caliber of blood vessels).

vibration.

(L. *vibrare,* to vibrate; pp. *vibratus*) vibrat-; vibrato-; vibro-.
Ex: vibrat-ile (vibrating or capable of vibrating); vibrato-genous (caused by vibration); vibro-therapeutics (the use of vibration in treatment of disease).

vibration (quiver).

(Gr. *pallein,* to shake) pall-; palle-.
Ex: pall-esthesia (the perception of vibratory movements); pall-anesthesia (loss of ability to perceive vibration); palle-genic (causing vibration).

viewing (examining; observing).

    (Gr. *skopein,* to view) -scope; -scopy; scopo-.

    Ex: fluoro-scope (a type of x-ray apparatus); micro-scope; endo-scope (an instrument used to examine the interior of an organ); cysto-scope (an instrument used to examine the interior of the bladder); opthalmo-scope (an instrument used to examine the eye); laryngo-scopy (examination of the larynx); scopo-philia (a keen desire to see sexual organs, or to show one's own); scopo-phobia (an abnormal aversion for bodily exposure).

villus (tuft).

    (L. *villus,* tuft) vill-; villi-; villus-.

    Ex: vill-itis (inflammation of a villus); villi-kinin (a hormone which stimulates the villi of the intestine); vill-ose (marked by the presence of villi); villus-ectomy (excision of a villus from a synovial membrane).

vinegar. See under *acid.*

virgin (virginity).

    (Gr. *parthenos,* virgin) parthen-; partheno-.

    Ex: partheno-genesis (production of offspring by virgin females, without involvement of spermatozoa); partheno-logy (the study of virginity or virgins); partheno-plasty (a plastic operation on the hymen to give a semblance of virginity); partheno-philia (a condition in which the male is interested only in a virgin female).

virus.

    (L. *virus,* poison) -vir-; viro-; virul-; viruli-.

    Ex: vir-al (pertaining to a virus); viro-genetic (caused by a virus); viro-logy (the study of viruses); viruli-cidal (capable of destroying a virus).

viscera (viscus; organ).

    (Gr. *splanchnos,* viscus) splanchn-; splanchnic-; splanchnico-; splanchno-.

    Ex: splanchn-ectopia (the presence of a viscus in an abnormal place); splanchnic-ectomy (excision of a viscus or the splanchnic nerve); splanchnico-tomy (the surgical cutting of a splanchnic nerve); splanchno-logy (the study of the viscera). See also *viscus.*

viscus (viscera).

(L. *viscus,* organ; pl. *viscera*) viscer-; visceri-; viscero-.

Ex: viscer-algia (pain in the viscera); visceri-motor (concerned with motor nerve impulses to a viscus or viscera); viscero-pleural (pertaining to viscera and the pleura); viscero-ptosis (a sagging of viscera).

visible (open; manifest; apparent).

(Gr. *phaneros,* visible) phaner-; phanero-.

Ex: phanero-genetic (of known origin or cause); phaner-osis (the process of becoming visible); phanero-philia (fondness for bodily exposure).

vision.

(L. *videre,* to see; pp. *visus*) vis-; visual-; visuo-.

Ex: vis-ible; visual-ization (act of making visible); visual-ize; visuo-gnosis (perception of visual impressions); visuo-psychic (both visual and psychic).

vision (condition of vision).

(Gr. *opsis,* sight) -opsia.

Ex: an-opsia (defective vision due to disuse); eu-opsia (normal condition of vision); hypochromat-opsia (condition in which colors appear pale); cyan-opsia (condition in which objects appear blue); heter-opsia (inequality of vision in the two eyes).

vision (eye; optic).

(Gr. *optos,* visible) opto-.

Ex: opto-gram (a visual image formed on the retina); opto-metry (the art of measuring the refraction of the eye); opto-type (a test type used in measuring vision).

vision (sight).

(Gr. *opsis,* sight) -opsis.

Ex: stere-opsis (vision in three dimensions); ent-opsis (visual sensation arising within the eye); Ambly-opsis (a genus of blind fish).

vision defect (defect of eye).

(Gr. *ops,* eye; genit. *opos*) -opia.

Ex: presby-opia (defective vision characteristic of the aged); my-opia (nearsightedness); hyper-opia (farsightedness); ametr-opia (defective refraction of the eye).

vitality. See under *life.*

vitamin.

(L. vita, life; amine) -vitamin-; vitamino-.

Ex: hypo-vitamin-osis (condition resulting from deficiency of vitamins in diet); pro-vitamin (a precursor of a vitamin); a-vitamin-osis; vitamino-genic (producing vitamins); vitamino-logy (the study of vitamins).

voice sound. See under *sound.*

vulva.

(L. *vulva,* covering) vulv-; vulvi-; vulvo-.

Ex: vulv-ar (pertaining to the vulva); vulv-itis (inflammation of the vulva); vulvo-crural (pertaining to the vulva and the thighs); vulvo-vaginal (pertaining to the vulva and the vagina).

W

walk (step).

(L. *gradi,* walk) grad-; gradi-; -grade.

Ex: gradi-genous (caused by walking); gradi-phobia (an aversion for walking); dys-grad-ia (difficult walking); digiti-grade (walking on the toes); planti-grade (walking on the entire sole of the foot).

wall. See under *septum.*

wall of organ (wall of body cavity).

(L. *paries,* wall; genit. *parietis*) pariet-; parieto-.

Ex: pariet-itis (inflammation of the wall of an organ or of the body); parieto-visceral (pertaining to the wall of a body cavity and the organs within the cavity).

warmth. See under *heat.*

wasting (withering; pulmonary tuberculosis).

(Gr. *phthiein,* to waste away) phthisic-; phthisio-.

Ex: phthisic-al (pertaining to pulmonary tuberculosis; marked by a wasting away); phthisio-phobia (fear of phthisis); phthisio-therapy (the treatment of phthisis).

water (fluid; hydrogen).

(Gr. *hydor,* water) hydr-; hydro-.

Ex: hydr-agogue (producing a watery stool); hydr-amnios (presence of excess of amniotic fluid); hydr-arthrosis (presence of fluid in a joint); hydro-carbon (compound containing hydrogen and carbon); hydro-cephalus (excess of fluid in the ventricles of the brain); an-hydr-ous (deprived of water).

wax (beeswax).

(L. *cera,* wax) cer-; cera-; cero-.

Ex: cer-aceous (waxy); cer-ate (ointment containing wax); cer-oma (tumor having a waxy consistency); cero-plasty (the making of anatomical models from wax); cer-umen (ear wax).

web. See under *tissue.*

wedge. See under *sphenoid bone.*

weight (pressure).

(Gr. *baros,* weight) bar-; baro-.

Ex: bar-agnosis (inability to appreciate the weight of objects); baro-meter (instrument for measuring atmospheric pressure); baro-trauma (injury caused by pressure).

well. See under *good.*

whip (whip-like process; flagellum).

(L. *flagellum,* whip) flagell-; flagelli-; flagello-.

Ex: flagell-ate (having a whip-like process; to whip); flagelli-form (shaped like a flagellum or whip); flagello-spore (a spore having a flagellum).

white.

(L. *albus,* white) alb-; albi-; albo-; albu-.

Ex: alb-ation (abnormal whitening); alb-in-ism (congenital absence of normal pigmentation); albi-genic (causing whiteness); albo-cinereous (pertaining to white and gray matter); albu-ginea (a white layer of fibrous tissue covering a structure).

white (white blood cell).

(Gr. *leukos,* white) leuc-; leuk-; leuko-.

Ex: leuc-ine (an amino acid); leuk-emia; leuko-cyte (white blood cell); leuko-penia (decrease in the number of white blood cells).

white blood cell. See under *white* and *leukocyte.*

whole. See under *entire.*

wide (broad).

> (Gr. *eurys,* wide) eury-.
>
> *Ex*: eury-cephalic (having a wide head); eury-gnathic (having a wide jaw); eury-thermic (capable of growing in a wide range of temperatures); eury-pelvic (having a wide pelvis).

wide (broad; flat).

> (Gr. *platys,* broad) platy-.
>
> *Ex*: platy-cephalic (having a wide head); platy-helminth (one of the flatworms); platy-rrhine (having a wide nose); platy-pellic (having a wide pelvis).

wing (wing-like structure; pterygoid process).

> (Gr. *pterygion,* wing) pterig-; pterigo-.
>
> *Ex*: pteryg-oid (shaped like a wing); pterygo-maxillary (pertaining to the pterygoid process and the maxilla); pterygo-palatine (pertaining to the pterygoid process and the palate).

with (together; at the same time; united).

> (Gr. *syn,* with) syn-; syl- (before letter *l*); sym- (before *m, p,* or *b*); sys- (before *s*).
>
> *Ex*: syn-chronism (occurrence at the same time); syn-dactyly (a growing together of adjacent digits); syn-drome (a group of signs and symptoms occurring together); sym-physis (a growing together); sys-tole (a drawing together; contraction).

with (together; in association).

> (L.) co- (before *w, h,* and all vowels); com- (before *b, p,* and *m*); con- (before *c, d, g, j, n, q, s, t, v*); col (before *l*); cor- (before *r*).
>
> *Ex*: co-arctate (press together); co-hesive (sticking together); com-patible (suitable for existence together); com-press (squeeze together); con-cresence (a growing together); con-fluent (flowing together); con-jugate (working together); col-lateral (working with another); cor-responding (in agreement with another).

withering. See under *wasting.*

within (inner; inside).

> (Gr. *entos,* inside) ent-; ento-.
>
> *Ex*: Ent-amoeba (a genus of amebas parasitic in the intestine); ent-epicondyle (the inner epicondyle); ento-derm (the inner-

most of the three layers of the embryo); ento-cele (an internal hernia).

within   (inner; inside; situated within).

(Gr. *endon,* within) end-; endo-.

Ex: end-arteritis (inflammation of the inner coat of an artery); end-emic (present within a community at all times); endo-cardium (membrane lining inner surface of the heart); endo-cranial (situated within the cranium); endo-thelium (layer of cells lining the inner surface of the heart, blood vessels, etc.).

within.   See under *in, inside, into,* and *inward.*

without   (not; absence; separation from; negative).

(L.) a- (before a consonant); an- (before a vowel).

Ex: a-bacterial (without bacteria); a-biotic (marked by absence of life); a-brachia (anomaly marked by absence of arms); a-geusia (lack of sense of taste); a-dynamia (absence of power); a-menorrhea (absence of menstruation); an-acidity (lack of acid-ity); an-esthesia (absence of sensation); an-orexia (absence of appetite). See also *not* and *out.*

woman   (female).

(Gr. *gyne,* woman; genit. *gynaikos*) gyn-; gyne-; gyno-; gyneco-.
Ex: gyn-andrism (a form of pseudohermaphroditism in the female); gyne-phobia (fear of, or aversion for, women); gyno-plasty (plastic surgery on the female sexual organs); gyneco-mastia (excessive development of the male breast).

womb.   See under *uterus.*

wood.

(Gr. *xylon,* wood) xylo-; xyl-.
Ex: xylo-carpous (bearing woody fruit); xylo-phagous (eating wood); xylo-plastic (pertaining to casts made of wood); xyl-ose (a kind of nonfermentable sugar).

word   (speech; discourse).

(Gr. *logos,* word) log-; logo-.
Ex: log-agnosia (inability to transmit ideas by language or words); logo-mania (excessive talkativeness); logo-plegia (pa-ralysis of the structures involved in speaking).

word.   See under *name.*

work (exertion; toil).

(Gr. *ponos,* toil) pono-.

Ex: pono-genous (caused by hard work); pono-philous (fond of work); pono-phobia (fear of hard work); pono-metry (measurement of exertion).

work (labor; energy).

(Gr. *ergon,* work; *ergasia,* labor) erg-; ergas-; ergasi-; ergasio-; ergo-.

Ex: ergasi-dermatosis (occupational dermatosis); ergasio-phobia (fear of work); ergo-graph (instrument used to record the work done by a muscle).

worm.

(L. vermis, worm) vermi-.

Ex: vermi-cide (a substance which destroys worms); vermi-cular (resembling a worm); vermi-fuge (a substance which expels worms); vermi-phobia (fear of worms).

worm (parasitic worm; intestinal worm).

(Gr. *helmins,* worm; genit. *helminthos*) helminth-; helminthi-; helmintho-.

Ex: helminth-agogue (a medicinal substance which expels parasitic worms); helminth-iasis (infestation with parasitic worms); helminthi-cide (a substance which kills parasitic worms); helmintho-logy (the science dealing with worms). See also *earthworm.*

write (describe; record).

(Gr. *graphein,* to write) -graph-; grapho-; -graphy.

Ex: a-graph-ia (loss of the ability to write); electrocardiograph; grapho-catharsis (release of emotional tensions through writing); grapho-motor (pertaining to the muscular movements involved in writing); radio-graphy (the making of x-ray pictures).

writing. See under *tracing.*

wrong. See under *improper.*

XYZ

xiphoid process.

(Gr. *xiphos,* sword) xiphi-; xipho-; xiphoid-.

Ex: xiphi-sternum (xiphoid process); xipho-costal (pertaining to the xiphoid process and the ribs); xiphoid-itis (inflammation of the xiphoid process); xipho-pagus (conjoined twins fused at the xiphoid process).

x-rays. See under *roentgen.*

yellow.

(Gr. *xanthos,* yellow) xanth-; xantho-.

Ex: xanth-emia (the presence of a yellow pigment in the blood); xantho-chromia (a yellowish discoloration); xantho-derma (yellowness of the skin); xantho-phyll (a yellow pigment of plants).

yellow (pale; pale yellow).

(Gr. *ochros,* pale yellow) ochro-.

Ex: ochro-dermia (a condition in which the skin is pale yellow); ochro-meter; ochro-nosis (a disease marked by a discoloration of certain tissues); ochro-dontia (yellowish discoloration of the teeth).

yellow (yellowness).

(L. *flavus,* yellow) flav-; flavi-; flavo-.

Ex: flav-aniline (a yellow dye); flav-escent (turning yellow); flavi-cant (yellowish); flavo-xanthin (yellow pigment).

yoke (connecting structure).

(L. *jugum,* yoke) jug-.

Ex: jug-ate (joined together); con-jug-al (pertaining to marriage); A-jug-a (a genus of herbs).

yolk.

(L. *vitellus,* yoke) -vitell-; vitello-; vitelli-.

Ex: micro-vitell-ine (having a small yolk); vitell-ary (pertaining to yolk); vitello-genesis (production of yolk); vitelli-coline (thriving in yolk).

yolk of an egg.

(Gr. *lekithos,* yolk) lecith-; lechitho-;

Ex: lecith-al (pertaining to, or having, a yolk); lecith-in; lecitho-vitellin (a suspension of egg yolk).

young child. See under *infant.*

zygoma (zygomatic arch; zygomatic bone; zygomatic process).
(Gr. *zygoma,* bar; *zygon,* yolk) zygomat-; zygomatico-.
Ex: zygomat-ic (pertaining to the zygoma); zygomatico-facial
(pertaining to the zygoma and the face); zygomatico-maxillary
(pertaining to the zygomatic bone and the maxillary bone).

zygomatic arch. See under *zygoma.*

zygomatic bone. See under *zygoma.*

APPENDIX

The following list contains the more common suffixes associated with the medical and other biological vocabularies. These abstract elements carry no specific ideas, but are the vectors of general concepts. Thus, a noun-forming suffix may designate *a condition, state, process, agency, or person performing a certain function.* An adjective-forming suffix may mean *able to, marked by, of the nature of, or like.* Each entry in the list gives the etymology of the suffix, its general meaning, and examples of its application.

-able (L. *-abilis*). An adjective-forming suffix meaning *able to, suitable for, characterized by,* or *capable of being. Ex:* operable; pot-able; palp-able; dialyz-able.

-ac (L. *-acus*). 1. An adjective-forming suffix meaning *characteristic of, pertaining to,* or *affected by. Ex:* hemophili-ac; cardi-ac. 2. A noun-forming suffix designating *a person affected by a specified condition. Ex:* mani-ac.

-acy (L. *-acia*). A suffix used to form nouns denoting *condition, quality,* or *status. Ex:* lun-acy; celib-acy.

-age (L. *-aticum*). A suffix forming nouns, usually from verbs, meaning an *act, state,* etc. *Ex:* drain-age; pass-age; dot-age.

-al (L. *-alis*). 1. An adjective-forming suffix meaning *pertaining to, having the characteristics of. Ex:* maniac-al; hysteric-al. 2. A noun-forming suffix meaning *a thing having a particular characteristic. Ex:* anim-al; perenni-al.

-ant (L. *-antem*). 1. An adjective-forming suffix meaning *having the characteristics of. Ex:* paralyz-ant; resist-ant. 2. A noun-forming suffix designating *one who* or *that which. Ex:* descend-ant; fumig-ant.

-ar (L. *-aris*). An adjective-forming suffix meaning *like,* or *of the nature of. Ex:* fil-ar; fibrill-ar; regul-ar.

-arium (L. *-arium*). A noun-forming suffix denoting *a place used for. Ex:* sol-arium; sanit-arium.

-ary (L. *-arius*). A suffix used to form nouns meaning *a person employed as, a thing used for,* etc. *Ex:* apothec-ary; diction-ary; formul-ary.

-ary (L. *-arius*). An adjective forming suffix meaning *pertaining to, connected with. Ex:* heredit-ary; volunt-ary; prim-ary.

-asis (L. *-asis*). A noun-forming suffix denoting *a condition, condition marked by. Ex*: schist-asis; psori-asis.

-ate (L. *-atus*). An adjective-forming suffix meaning *characterized by, shaped like. Ex*: flagell-ate; umbilic-ate; genicul-ate; turbin-ate.

-ate (L. *-ate*). A verb-forming suffix meaning *to become, to produce, to treat with. Ex*: evapor-ate; invagin-ate; conjug-ate; prolifer-ate; ulcer-ate; vaccin-ate; chlorin-ate; indur-ate.

-ate (L. *-atus*). A noun-forming suffix designating a *person or thing having a certain status. Ex*: diplom-ate; candid-ate.

-ation (L. *-ation*). A suffix used to form nouns denoting *a process, action,* or *condition. Ex*: gyr-ation; agglutin-ation; inactiv-ation.

-cy (L. *-cia*). A noun-forming suffix denoting *a condition, status,* or *fact of being. Ex*: normal-cy; infan-cy; idio-cy.

-ent (L. *-ens*; *-entis*). 1. An adjective-forming suffix meaning *characterized by, having the quality of, performing the action of. Ex*: incongru-ent; conflu-ent. 2. A noun-forming suffix designating *one who* or *that which. Ex*: absorb-ent; superintend-ent.

-eous (L. *-eus*). An adjective-forming suffix meaning *like,* or *of the nature of. Ex*: aqu-eous; vitr-eous; nacr-eous.

-er (L. *arius*). A noun-forming suffix indicating *a person or thing performing a given activity. Ex*: lexicograph-er; urethre-urynt-er.

-escence (L. *-escens*). A noun-forming suffix indicating *a process, act of becoming, etc. Ex*: biolumin-escence; phosphor-escence.

-escent (L. *-escens; -escentis*). A verb-forming suffix meaning *in the process of, becoming, beginning to be, etc. Ex*: flav-escent; conval-escent.

-esis (Gr. *-esis*). A noun-forming suffix denoting *a process, action, etc. Ex*: cataphor-esis.

-etic (Gr. *-etikos*). An adjective-forming suffix denoting *a quality, characteristic, feature. Ex*: polyphyl-etic; gen-etic; pyr-etic.

-fy (L. *facere*). A verb-making suffix meaning *to make, to cause, cause to become. Ex*: lique-fy; emulsi-fy; magni-fy; rare-fy.

-ia (L. *-ia*). A noun-forming suffix used in *names of diseases, names of biological classes.* Ex: Pneumon-ia; hyster-ia; hemophil-ia; hematur-ia; Amphib-ia; Mammal-ia.

-ible (L. *-ibilis*). An adjective-forming suffix meaning *capable of being, able to.* Ex: refrang-ible; combust-ible; digest-ible.

-ic (L. *-icus*). An adjective-forming suffix meaning *of, pertaining to, characteristic of.* Ex: organ-ic; protoplasm-ic; alcohol-ic; cephal-ic; podal-ic; somat-ic.

-ical (L. *-icalis*). An adjective-forming suffix indicating a *quality, characteristic.* Ex: physiolog-ical; patholog-ical.

-icity (L. *-icitas*). A noun-forming suffix denoting a *quality,* or *condition.* Ex: organ-icity; chron-icity; eccentr-icity; pathogen-icity.

-id (L. *-idus*). An adjective-forming suffix denoting *a quality,* or *characteristic.* Ex: rab-id; fet-id; orch-id.

-ile (L. *-ilis*). A noun-forming and adjective-forming suffix designating *suitability, quality,* or *relationship with.* Ex: lab-ile; frag-ile; juven-ile; vir-ile.

-ility (L. *-ilitas*). A noun-forming suffix denoting *a condition, state,* etc. Ex: curab-ility; sensib-ility; susceptib-ility.

-ion (L. *-io*; genit. *-ionis*). A suffix forming nouns, chiefly from verbs, indicating an *act, process, condition,* or *state.* Ex: incis-ion; infus-ion; lacerat-ion.

-ism (L. *-ismus*). A noun-forming suffix designating *an act, process, condition, action.* Ex: hermaphrodit-ism; cocain-ism; digital-ism; dicrot-ism; hypnot-ism; alcohol-ism; infantil-ism.

-ismus (L. *-ismus*). A noun-forming suffix indicating *an abnormal condition.* Ex: tr-ismus; sphincter-ismus.

-ist (L.-*ista*). A suffix forming nouns which denote *a person engaged in a certain occupation, person skilled in a given field.* Ex: pharmac-ist; chem-ist; gynecolog-ist; orthoped-ist.

-itic (L. *-iticus*). An adjective-forming suffix meaning *caused by, of the nature of.* Ex: syphil-itic; arthr-itic.

-itious (L. *-itius*). An adjective-forming suffix meaning *characterized by, of the nature of.* Ex: icter-itious; nutr-itious.

-ity (L. *-itas*). A suffix forming nouns denoting *a condition, state, character.* Ex: multipar-ity; steril-ity.

-ive (L. *-ivus*). An adjective-forming suffix meaning *pertaining to, of, having the quality of, tending to. Ex*: suppurat-ive; refract-ive; ulcerat-ive.

-ization (L. *-izare*). A suffix used to form nouns from verbs, denoting *a process, condition, act. Ex*: fertil-ization; immun-ization.

-ize (L. *-izare*). A verb-forming suffix meaning *cause to be, become, treat with, subject to, combine with. Ex*: steril-ize; oxid-ize; iod-ize; fertil-ize.

-or (L. *-or*). A noun-forming suffix denoting *a person or thing performing* a particular function; also, or *a condition, quality. Ex*: don-or; respirat-or; pall-or.

-ory (L. *-orius*). A suffix forming adjectives meaning *having the nature of, of, pertaining to,* or *serving for. Ex*: secret-ory; ambulat-ory; access-ory; incis-ory; saltat-ory; refract-ory.

-ory (L. *-orium*). A suffix forming nouns meaning *a place for, a thing for,* or *that which serves for. Ex*: laborat-ory; cremat-ory; reposit-ory.

-ose (L. *-osus*). An adjective-forming suffix meaning *provided with, having,* or *like. Ex*: comat-ose; ram-ose; varic-ose; rug-ose; ventr-ose.

-ose (F. *-ose*). A noun-forming suffix indicating *a sugar, carbohydrate, product of protein hydrolysis. Ex*: sucr-ose; levul-ose; cellul-ose; album-ose.

-osis (Gr. *-osis*). A suffix forming nouns denoting *action, condition, disorder,* or *abnormal condition. Ex*: lord-osis; kyph-osis; neur-osis; osm-osis; avitamin-osis.

-otic (Gr. *-otikos*). A suffix used to form adjectives meaning *pertaining to, affected with, causing,* or *producing. Ex*: neur-otic; osm-otic; hypn-otic; scler-otic.

-ous (L. *-osus*). An adjective-forming suffix meaning *characterized by, having,* or *having a lower valence. Ex*: contagi-ous; polymorph-ous; ferr-ous.

-sis (Gr. *-esis*). A suffix forming nouns denoting *a condition, activity. Ex*: peristal-sis.

-tion (L. *-tio; -tionis*). A noun-forming suffix meaning *act, process, condition,* or *state. Ex*: ablacta-tion.

-ule (L. *-ulus*). A noun-forming suffix indicating *diminutive size, smallness.* *Ex*: pap-ule; phlycten-ule; gran-ule; ov-ule; ven-ule.

-ulent (L. *-ulentus*). An adjective-forming suffix meaning *full of, containing.* *Ex*: corp-ulent; pur-ulent.

-ure (L. *-ura*). A suffix forming nouns meaning *result of an action, agent, instrumentality* *Ex*: junct-ure; ligat-ure; punct-ure.

-y (L. *-ia*). A suffix forming nouns denoting *condition, quality.* *Ex*: heredit-y; obesit-y; allerg-y.